TEXTBOOK OF
Bloodbanking Science

TEXTBOOK OF
Bloodbanking Science

Chester M. Zmijewski, PH.D.
Associate Professor, Pathology
University of Pennsylvania School of Medicine
Director, Immunology Laboratory
Division of Laboratory Medicine
Hospital of the University of Pennsylvania
Philadelphia, Pennsylvania

and

Walter E. Haesler, Jr., M.S., MT (ASCP) SBB
Lecturer Immunohematology
University of Pennsylvania School of Medicine
Technical Supervisor
Blood Transfusion Service
Division of Laboratory Medicine
Hospital of the University of Pennsylvania
Philadelphia, Pennsylvania

APPLETON-CENTURY-CROFTS/NEW YORK

82 83 84 85 86 / 10 9 8 7 6 5 4 3 2 1

Prentice-Hall International, Inc., London
Prentice-Hall of Australia, Pty. Ltd., Sydney
Prentice-Hall of India Private Limited, New Delhi
Prentice-Hall of Japan, Inc., Tokyo
Prentice-Hall of Southeast Asia (Pte.) Ltd., Singapore
Whitehall Books Ltd., Wellington, New Zealand

Library of Congress Cataloging in Publication Data

Zmijewski, Chester M.
    Blood banking science.

Bibliography: p.
    Includes index.
    1. Blood banks.   2. Blood—Collection and preservation.
I. Haesler, Walter E.   II. Title.
RM172.Z58   615'.39   81-20557
ISBN 0-8385-8869-7   AACR2

Cover and text design: Jean M. Sabato

Production editor: Ina J. Shapiro

PRINTED IN THE UNITED STATES OF AMERICA

CONTENTS

PREFACE

In preparing this text we have attempted to gear our remarks to an audience who is approaching the clinical aspect of medical technology for the first time. Therefore the major focus is on general principles and overall operational procedures. This has not been an easy task. Over the years we have naturally succumbed to favoritism with respect to certain specialized areas and brushed aside those aspects that, although important, are only of peripheral personal interest. Even though we have made a genuine effort to avoid giving our own specialities an unfairly large amount of attention, this has not been always possible. For this we apologize. However, in spite of this, we sincerely hope that the underlying message will be clear. We have developed a certain fondness for this discipline and hope some of the resultant enthusiasm will pass on to the students who read this book.

Finally, we would like to extend our sincere appreciation to the many friends who have helped in the preparation of this work. Special thanks are due to Dr. Emanuel Hackel, who helped focus the section on genetics, Chris Zmijewski, who prepared the illustrations, and Diane Stevenson, who typed the manuscript.

CHAPTER 1

Introduction and Historical Aspects

Objectives

The information presented in this chapter should enable the student to:

1. Understand the relationship of the blood bank to the clinical laboratory as a whole.
2. Describe the role of the technologist in the blood bank laboratory.
3. Define the problems that had to be solved before transfusion could become a routine therapeutic reality.
4. Describe Denis's account of a transfusion reaction.
5. Relate the events leading up to the establishment of the first blood bank.
6. Appreciate the contribution of plastic blood bags to the modern practice of transfusion therapy.

From a technologist's point of view, the blood bank traditionally has been one of the most challenging of all of the clinical laboratories. This is one of the few laboratories that as yet has not been invaded by highly sophisticated but otherwise impersonal automated equipment. In this laboratory, perhaps more so than in any other, the technologists' skills are taxed to their fullest and each worker has an opportunity to experience a true medical relationship with the patient.

One of the reasons for the closeness that exists between the laboratory worker and patient in this particular field is that the administration of a mismatched or improperly tested unit of blood can result in a severe reaction or even death. Because of this awesome realization, some technologists may go so far as to develop a fear of the blood bank laboratory. This is totally uncalled for, since modern systems that are constantly being improved are designed to protect the patient. Nevertheless, while it need not be feared, blood banking should be respected. Meticulous attention must be afforded to clerical and technical details, which is what makes this field so challenging.

Finally, the blood bank laboratory is one of the few remaining laboratories where a technologist working at the bench is in a position to make discoveries that are of potentially important scientific impact. Most of the new findings that have contributed substantially to our fuller understanding of the behavior and inheritance of blood group antigens have been possible because of the keen observations of technologists. The anticipation of potential discovery, of itself, can make this a challenging and rewarding career.

Today, the use of whole blood is a well-accepted and commonly employed measure without which many modern surgical procedures could not be carried out. The historical development of this therapeutic modality is fascinating, a brief synopsis of which will serve as a fitting introduction to the field.

Blood has always held a mysterious fascination for people and traditionally was thought of as being the living force of the body. Historians tell us that the ancient Egyptians, cognizant of the beneficial and lifegiving properties of blood, used it for baths to resuscitate the sick and rejuvenate the old and incapacitated. In ancient Rome, spectators rushed into the arena to drink the blood of dying gladiators. They believed that this blood was especially beneficial because the athletes were strong and brave, qualities that were located in and transmissible by their blood.

In the middle ages, the drinking of blood was advocated as a tonic for rejuvenation and the treatment of various diseases.[1] In the summer of 1492 the blood of three robust young boys was given to the ailing Pope Innocent VIII (Fig. 1). Apparently the procedure was not successful, since it is recorded that the Pope died on July 25, 1492. Unfortunately, this particular therapeutic regimen was even more devastating since the three youths also died as a result of their donation.

Traditionally it is accepted that Adreas Libavius was the first to advocate a blood transfusion, in 1615. The method he described was essentially a direct transfusion, but most historians seriously doubt that he actually attempted his experimental procedure. Harvey's treatise on the circulation of blood added impetus to the investigation of intravenous therapy, which resulted in a flurry of reports during the early 1600s.

One of the pioneers of the authentic practice of transfusion was Richard

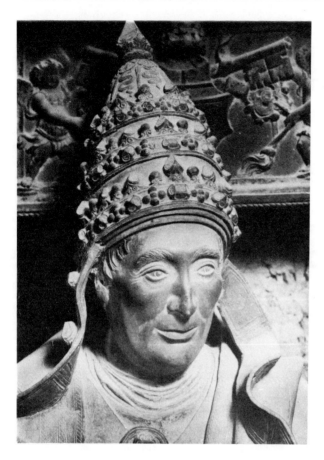

Fig. 1. Pope Innocent VIII, one of the first recorded recipients of a blood draught. (*From Brusher,* Popes Through the Ages. *Courtesy of Borden Publishing Company.*)

Lower, an English physician, who performed his experiments on dogs in 1665. His account of the procedure is the first description of a direct transfusion from artery to vein. According to Lower, a small dog was exsanguinated from the jugular vein until he was almost dead. Then a quill was connected to the cervical artery of a large donor dog, and the blood allowed to flow until the recipient was "overfilled and burdened by the amount of the inflowing blood." The procedure was repeated several times, after which the recipient dog's condition returned to normal. In subsequent experiments Lower substituted specially designed silver tubes for the quills originally employed as a means of anastomosing the circulation of the two animals (Fig. 2). During the next several years similar studies were repeated in England and in France. The investigators, however, began to vary their techniques somewhat; they attempted exchanges of small amounts of blood between animals of different species. Eventually, of course, their thoughts turned to humans.

A short time later, Lower and King transfused sheep blood into people. The way these experiments were performed was often diagrammed in textbooks of the day. One such illustration, from Scultetus in 1693[2] (Fig. 3), shows a man being transfused with the blood of a dog. A puncture has been made in the subject's arm

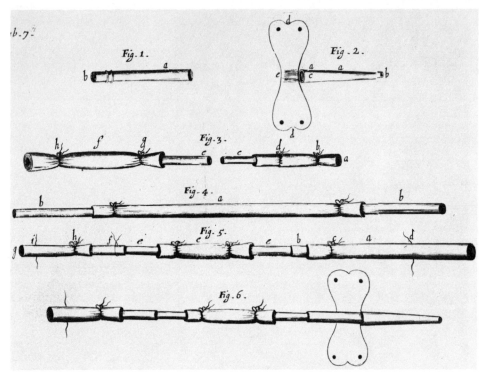

Fig. 2. Silver cannulae designed by Lower for performing direct blood transfusions in dogs. (*Courtesy of Trent Collection, Duke University Medical Center Library.*)

from which the blood rushes geiserlike into a basin, probably to make room for the blood flowing in from the dog. This concept was in keeping with the original method used by Lower when transfusing dogs.

In 1667, Jean Denis, physician to Louis XIV, transfused a small amount of blood from a lamb into the vein of a young man suffering from leutic madness. The technique was successful, although he wrote that following the transfusion, the patient passed urine as black as soot, but apparently there was little effect on either his good physical state or his poor mental one.

After his initial success, Denis continued his experiments on other patients. Unfortunately, the fourth patient in his series died. Denis's description of this particular case indicated that the patient in question was suffering from syphilis and had been transfused twice before. The first infusion of blood produced no detectable symptoms. The second time, however, "his arm became hot, the pulse rose, sweat burst out over his forehead, he complained of pain in the kidneys and was sick at the bottom of his stomach. The urine was very dark, in fact, black." After the third transfusion the patient died. This description is probably the first recorded account of the signs and symptoms of what is recognized today as a hemolytic transfusion reaction. The most likely explanation for its absence in the previous in-

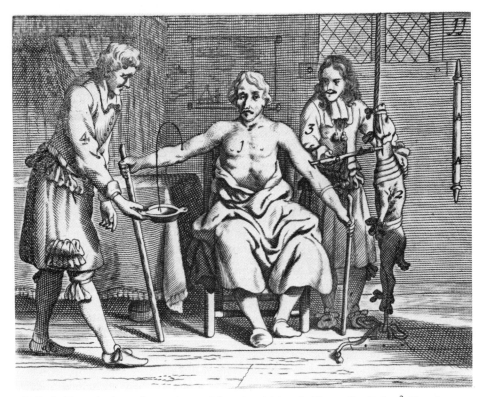

FIG. 3. Transfusion of a patient with animal blood. (*From Scultetus.*[2] *Courtesy of the National Library of Medicine.*)

stances is that the volumes of blood were relatively small and the symptoms benign enough to go unnoticed. As a result of this unfortunate outcome, the patient's wife charged Denis with murder. A long legal battle ensued. Eventually, Denis was exonerated of the murder charge, but the courts decreed that transfusions were to be prohibited except with the sanction of the Faculty of Medicine of Paris. Several years later, an edict of the British Parliament similarly prohibited transfusions and drew an official close to the first phase of man's desire to replace the vital force of the body.

The actual practice of transfusion lay dormant for nearly 150 years, although the basic idea did not escape the minds of the scientific community. As medical knowledge advanced, physicians began to understand the real importance of blood, not merely as a mysterious tonic or rejuvenating potion, but as an essential material with a physiologic function that made it a requirement for life.

Although some claim that a Dr. Philip Syng, Physic of Philadelphia, performed a transfusion as early as 1795[3] many stories have been written about one particular English obstetrician, James Blundell. It has been said that he was appalled at his own helplessness at combatting fatal hemorrhage during delivery, and in 1818, he revived the procedure of blood transfusion.

It is apparent that Blundell's motivation stemmed from an idea that the loss of blood could be detrimental or even fatal. His research efforts extended to studying the effect of the withdrawal of various amounts of blood. This approach was founded on a new concept. No longer was the procedure based on mysticism and the ancient desire to replace old blood with new blood or to rid a suffering patient of evil humors. Instead, it was subjected to astute scientific investigation. Blundell and his collaborators performed a considerable number of experiments. They demonstrated the shocking effects of withdrawing large quantities of blood from an animal, much in the same manner as Lower did many years before. However, they also showed that these effects could be reversed with relatively small quantities of blood that were in no way injurious to the donor animal. This was an important observation, for it was certainly of no use to proceed with the development of a technique that might bring harm to a potential donor of blood.

Blundell performed ten transfusions, two of which were on patients who had already died. Of the total, four were successful. In all the cases human blood was used. This was indeed fortunate, otherwise a set of circumstances similar to those experienced by Denis would surely have been encountered. Blundell's experiments showed that when a dog was exsanguinated and subsequently transfused with the blood of another dog, it survived.[1] If, on the other hand, the contents of its circulatory system were replaced with blood from a sheep, the dog showed an initial recovery but invariably died. This indicated that species barriers had to be observed.

As a result of problems encountered with blood clotting, direct transfusions were most often employed using some very ingenious devices to speed up the flow of blood (Fig. 4). In 1914 and 1915, this problem was solved when Hustin, Agote, Lewisohn, and Wein and other investigators noted that small, nontoxic quantities of citrate prevented the coagulation of blood. In 1916, Rous and Turner discovered that the use of small amounts of dextrose added greatly to the preservation of the quality of blood undergoing storage.[4] These discoveries prompted Dr. Oswald Robertson to use transfusion of previously collected blood to treat severely wounded soldiers during the first world war.

Possibly as a direct result of the development of suitable anticoagulants and the discovery that blood maintained at 4C could be stored for up to ten days, as well as his own investigators' efforts, in 1937 Dr. Bernard Fantus established the

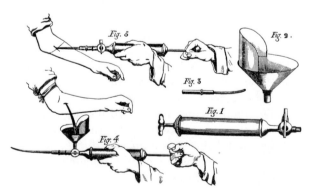

Fig. 4. Syringe designed by Waller to expedite direct transfusions. The blood was collected into the funnel and aspirated into the syringe. The stopcock was then rotated and the blood expelled into the recipient through the attached cannula. (*Courtesy of Trent Collection, Duke University Medical Center Library.*)

first blood bank in the world[5] at the Cook County Hospital in Chicago as the blood preservation laboratory. The first blood bank technologist was a pharmacist, Charles J. Mattas, and the first supervisor was Dr. Elizabeth Schirmer.

Fantus, being a far-sighted individual, coined the term *blood bank*. He reasoned that since a bank implies a system of deposits, savings, and withdrawals, it would be possible to establish a bioeconomic structure to serve the patients' needs. It is interesting to note that the concept of the paid donor originated in this first blood bank as well. As friends and relatives became too few to satisfy the needs, unrelated donors were paid for their efforts. Thus it may be said that Fantus's idea of a bank truly came to pass, since it suffered from the same woes that plague our financial banking institutions and he had to resort to the same economic tactics.

The ultimate anticoagulant and preservative that is in widespread use today was not described until 1943, by Loutit and Mollison.[6] The solution ACD (acid-citrate-dextrose) is capable of maintaining blood in a transfusable condition for twenty-one days at 4C. A newer solution, CPDA-1 (citrate-phosphate-dextrose with adenine), has been developed that will permit a refrigerator shelf life of up to thirty-one–five days. The whole idea of the blood bank, of course, is now widespread and has grown into a separate medical subspecialty of its own. Laboratories devoted to this area are located in every modern hospital throughout the world and donor collection centers exist in all major communities. Largely through the efforts of such organizations as the American Association of Blood Banks (AABB) and the American Red Cross (ARC), the public is accepting the fact that blood donation is a social obligation.

Another novel approach to transfusion was introduced by Shamov and Yudin,[7] Russian investigators who pioneered the use of cadaver blood for transfusion. This technique offers certain advantages in that anticoagulants are not required because of natural fibrinolysis, and large transfusions can be taken from a single donor. There are numerous disadvantages as well, however, including an adequate supply of suitable cadavers; that is, people who have died from causes other than septicemia, malignancy, or metabolic disease affecting the blood. Even though this method is very popular in Russia, it has never been used widely in this country.

The field of blood storage and preservation has been the subject of intensive investigation in recent years. Whereas at one time it was necessary to bring an animal or human donor into the bedchamber, it is now possible to collect blood at leisure, ship it across great distances, and even store it in the frozen state with the aid of certain solutions. In this manner large quantities of blood can be stockpiled for future use in the event of a disaster or other emergency.

The development of anticoagulants was a solution to only one of the problems that confronted the early therapists. The second problem was the violent and fatal sequelae that often occurred subsequent to blood transfusion. The first account of such a reaction was described earlier in this chapter. That particular reaction took place principally because animal blood was used for transfusion. Similar events, however, undoubtedly occurred even when human blood was used, and these account for the limited success reported by Blundell and others. We know today that these phenomena are the result of red cell destruction by immunologic mechanisms that take place because of the individual differences of human blood. This problem was not solved until after 1900 and was the stimulus for generating interest in an area that was to become the field of immunohematology.

The clinical practice of blood transfusion therapy has changed considerably over the years due to a number of factors, including increasing knowledge and the implementation of new technology. Whole blood is composed of several cellular and soluble elements, each with its own set of individual functions. As these functions were better understood through research, it became apparent that whole blood transfusions were not always necessary. Indeed, in some cases the use of whole blood when only a single element was required could produce deleterious effects. This led to the concept of blood component therapy. The most significant event that made this approach a reality was the development of plastic bags for the collection of whole blood.

Previously, blood had been collected in glass bottles of various configurations. Regardless of their design, however, they all had the same disadvantages. First, the closure was a rubber stopper that was inserted and sealed in at the time of manufacture. To allow blood to flow into this container at the time of donation, a vacuum was created inside the bottle. The blood therefore had to be collected by means of a vacuum, sometimes forcibly creating a situation that was dangerous to certain cellular elements. To collect the blood, a donor set had to be inserted through the rubber stopper, thus breaking the sterile factory seal and introducing bacterial contamination. If the blood were to be collected by gravity flow, the vacuum in the bottle had to be broken by a suitable airway, which had to be kept open during the donation to allow the displaced air to escape. Similarly, an airway had to be used during transfusion to permit air to displace the fluid in the rigid container. These airways were a general nuisance since they would become clogged, a condition leading to an undesirable and dangerous build-up of air pressure. Although centrifugation of these containers was possible, it often led to breakage, with subsequent loss of the unit. In addition, because of design, these containers could not be manipulated easily.

The plastic blood bag eliminates all of these difficulties. The donor tubing and collection needle are fused into the plastic bag at the time of manufacture. This eliminates possible contamination at the time of collection. Since the bag is made of flexible plastic and is manufactured as a collapsed container, there is no need to introduce airways to collect blood by gravity. The flexibility of the container readily allows it to adapt to changes in hydrostatic and atmospheric pressures as well as presenting less danger of breakage during centrifugation. Finally, the bags can be made in tandem so that the partial contents of one can be transferred to another without disturbing the integrity of the closed system. This allows for a number of different manipulations. Using different types of blood bags, one can prepare red cells for the treatment of anemia, platelets for bleeding disorders, and plasma factors for hemophilia from a single unit of blood. This permits not only a more efficient utilization of whole blood but also a far superior therapeutic regimen.

The need for the development of newer methods of component preparation has created new ideas in engineering. An entire generation of instruments devised for the collection and preparation of blood products is now on the market. Some of

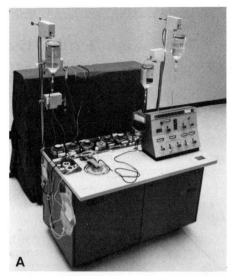

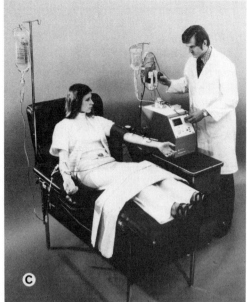

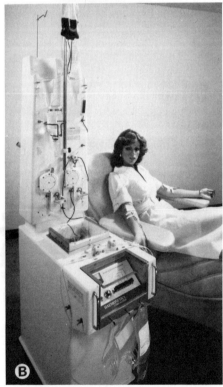

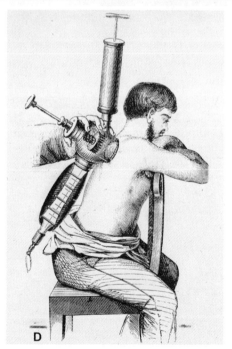

Fig. 5. Contemporary instruments used for the continuous-flow processing of blood components compared with an ancient device. **A.** IBM, **B.** Haemonetics, and **C.** Fenwal blood processors are connected in-line with the donor's blood flow. The blood is drawn into the machine, the components separated and collected, and the unwanted components returned to the donor. **D.** Instrument designed by Gesellius for obtaining capillary blood from donors, 1873. (*Photos courtesy of IBM, Princeton, NJ; Haemonetics Corp, Natick, Mass; Fenwal Labs, Morton-Grove, Ill; and the Trent Collection, Duke University Medical Center Library.*)

these, because of their size and complexity, are reminiscent of apparatus used early in transfusion history (Fig. 5).

The achievements possible with these devices, however, are remarkable: one can separate whole blood into red cells, platelets, plasma, and even white cells in a continuous closed system, permitting reinfusion of the donor with the unwanted product. In this manner, large numbers of platelets or leukocytes can be collected repeatedly from the same individual. Since the red cells are returned to the donor, the total circulating red cell mass is not depleted; therefore, platelets can be prepared from the same person several times a week with no harmful effects. This same system can also be used for such therapeutic purposes as plasmapheresis and even plasma exchange. Finally, devices are currently being investigated that can recycle blood that has been lost during major surgical procedures. The use of such devices would greatly reduce the total number of units of red cells needed from separate donors, thereby reducing the immunologic risks inherent in the exposure to a large number of foreign antigens.

REFERENCES

1. Keynes G: Blood Transfusion. Bristol, John Wright and Sons, Ltd, 1949.
2. Scultetus J: Armamentarium Chirugicum. Leyden, 1693.
3. Schmidt PJ: Transfusion in America in the eighteenth and nineteenth centuries. N Engl J Med 279:1319, 1968.
4. Oberman HA: Evolution of blood transfusion. Univ Mich Med Center J 33:68, 1967.
5. Telischi M: Evolution of Cook County Hospital Blood Bank. Transfusion 14:623, 1974.
6. Loutit JF and Mollison PL: Advantages of a disodium-citrate-glucose mixture as a blood preservative. Br Med J 2:744, 1943.
7. Yudin SS: Transfusion of cadaver blood. JAMA 106:997, 1936.

CHAPTER 2

Modern-Day Concepts

Objectives

By reading this chapter the student should learn the:
1. Operational aspects of a blood bank.
2. Differences and similarities between blood banks and financial savings banks.
3. Manner in which blood banks obtain and maintain a supply of blood.
4. Function of a transfusion service and its regulation.
5. Definition of a procedure manual.
6. Methods used to store and preserve whole blood.
7. Useful components of whole blood and general methods for their preparation.
8. Shelf life of blood components.
9. Principles of cryopreservation.

BLOOD BANK ADMINISTRATION

In recent years the field of blood bank administration has become an area of expertise in its own right. This has happened because the modern blood bank operates in some ways like a large enterprise engaged in the supply of a perishable, consumable product, the major difference being that the product cannot be manufactured and its use is dictated by medical circumstances that can be neither controlled nor accurately predicted.

Many of the larger blood banks, therefore, have turned for guidance to business professionals who have acquired specialized knowledge relating to blood bank operations. For this reason, the person interested in the medical technology of blood banking science rarely if ever needs to be overly concerned with the administrative aspects of the service. However, a rudimentary knowledge of the principles involved will help the bench technologist to appreciate some of the administrative problems, thereby creating a harmonious atmosphere for cooperation. Further, such information will be of invaluable aid in smaller operations where the blood bank technologists have multiple responsibilities.

Briefly, the service universally referred to as the blood bank is in reality two services. The first of these, and the one of most interest to the student of medical technology, is the transfusion service. This is the operation that selects appropriate units of blood for transfusion, i.e., units that will not harm the patient in any manner. The bulk of this text is devoted to the basic immunology principles and serologic methods by which this can be accomplished. The second part of the operation is the bank itself. This is the operation that collects units of blood that can be used for transfusion, maintains an adequate inventory to satisfy consumer demands, and provides some sort of system of debits and credits for its clientele.

Basically, a blood bank operates in the same fashion as any other bank. The depositors, or, in this case the blood donors, deposit units of blood in the bank. This blood is then used by the bank for the needs of the patients it serves. When the donors themselves or their designated representatives require a transfusion, it is the bank's responsibility to provide the blood. Unlike a financial bank, however, the blood bank must be a dynamic operation, dictated by the short shelf life of the product that mandates constant replenishment.

This rather simplistic approach is complicated by several factors, the most prominent of which is that, as will be seen from the remainder of this text, blood comes in eight different types and each patient must be transfused with his or her own type. On the other hand, the donors are random volunteers from the population at large. Therefore, the operator of the bank has no choice as to the type of blood that is deposited at any given time. Thus, fluctuation in the supply of the different types is inevitable. This is compensated for in part by recruiting enough donors to insure that all types will be adequately represented. Even so there will be times when an oversupply of some types and a shortage of other types will occur.

Another complication is that unexpected medical emergencies demanding extraordinarily large quantities of blood of a given type can deplete supplies very quickly. Obviously, a blood bank cannot operate efficiently all by itself. It needs to belong to a clearinghouse or system comparable to the Federal Reserve System that exists among financial banks, allowing blood inventories obtained by the individual banks to be adjusted and equilibrated to meet their needs. Units of the types that are in oversupply in one region can be transferred to the reserve system, through which they can be reassigned to those regions in which they are in short supply. Similarly, types of blood in short supply can be "borrowed" from the system.

Two such systems now operate throughout the United States under the auspices of the American Red Cross and the American Association of Blood Banks. Most hospital blood banks belong to one of these two systems and sometimes to both. Although the basic philosophies under which they operate differ in certain minor points, they both have a common goal, to provide blood of the specific type and in the quantity required to patients who need it, regardless of the dispensing location.

In some instances a third alternative is available in the form of a community blood center. Such a center accepts donations of blood from a large community, such as an entire large metropolitan area or perhaps even a portion of a state. Although such centers can draw on a large donor population to equilibrate supply with demand, they too find it convenient to be associated with one of the major systems.

Regardless of the approach, the provision of an adequate supply of blood is a community responsibility. Unfortunately, not all citizens of a community realize this, because they are healthy. Therefore, educating the population and instilling awareness is one of the predominant duties of blood bank administrators.

With these ideas in mind it is possible to begin to answer the basic question of where a hospital blood bank gets its donor blood. Three sources can be tapped. First of all, if the institution is large enough, it can collect its own volunteer donors and donors who are indebted to the bank because one of their relatives or friends may have received blood from the bank during a recent hospitalization. With additional effort such large institutions often operate predeposit plans, whereby people can come in and donate for their own, their family's, or their organization's members' future needs. Such banks frequently use the American Association of Blood Banks clearinghouse system to adjust their supplies. On the other hand, if the institution is not large enough to support its own donor program or if for some other reason it prefers to concentrate its efforts in areas other than donor procurement, it may subscribe either totally or in part to the services of the American Red Cross or some community blood center. The blood service organization provides a full inventory of blood of the various types to the hospital bank to the extent that its own resources will allow. As a third alternative, the hospital bank may purchase its blood from commercial blood banks, proprietary organizations that pay their donors for blood. Although in recent years the use of paid donors has been discouraged and in some states it is illegal to transfuse such blood unless the unit is plainly labeled, there are a number of respectable commercial banks. The reason for discouraging this practice is that a higher transmission incidence of posttransfusion hepatitis results from the use of paid donor blood than when blood from volunteers is used exclusively.

THE TRANSFUSION SERVICE

The modern transfusion service, or, more properly, the department of hemotherapy, is a complex organization. This department procures and provides whole blood and blood components for the patients it serves. Likewise, it provides the professional and technical knowledge that is required so that the maximum benefits are obtained by the patients to whom the blood is issued. In addition, the department is expected to provide the facilities, technical expertise, and equipment necessary to perform such therapeutic procedures as therapeutic phlebotomies and plasma-, platelet-, and leukapheresis on the request of the staff physicians. The department may also do serologic studies as aids in the diagnosis of autoimmune hemolytic anemia, perform prenatal studies to detect possible fetomaternal blood group incompatibility; and issue Rh_o immunoglobulin to prevent Rh alloimmunization.

Blood and its components are not only biological products but also drugs and as such can be dispensed only by a physician's prescription. In addition, since these items are drugs their manufacture (procurement) and disposition (either dispensed or discarded) are under the jurisdiction of the Bureau of Biologics (BOB) of the Food and Drug Administration (FDA), U.S. Department of Health and Human Services. This agency has extensive regulations governing the operational conduct of the department and are reflected in each laboratory's standard operating procedures manual. Since this manual must be updated annually and approved by the director of the facility, the document represents the precise interpretation of the federal regulations as they apply to the individual facility. Therefore, every medical technologist must be thoroughly familiar with its contents.

A good procedure manual will be indexed and contain the exact methods to be used in performing every test in the laboratory along with appropriate references. Among other things, it will contain statements of laboratory policy. For example, it should state the policy for the selection of blood for the transfusion of newborn infants or the procedures to follow when a transfusion reaction is suspected and reported. Finally, it should give the names of people to contact in an emergency.

Blood Storage and Preservation

Whole blood used for transfusion is a human tissue composed of metabolically active cellular elements and plasma containing enzymes, which will decompose unless properly cared for. To retard this natural tendency to decay, the blood is collected into an anticoagulant that provides nourishment for the cellular elements but provides a biochemical environment that appreciably lowers their metabolic rate. Several solutions are available for this purpose, including ACD (acid-citrate-dextrose) and CPD (citrate-phosphate-dextrose), which provide a shelf life of twenty-one days, and CPDA-1 (citrate-phosphate-dextrose with adenine). This latter solution contains the amino acid adenine to maintain adequate levels of the energy source ATP in addition to the nutrient dextrose and extends the shelf life of whole blood to thirty-five days. These dating periods, however, are valid only if the blood is continuously stored at $4C \pm 2C$. Refrigeration is critical and must be maintained exactly. If the temperature is too high, the metabolism will be accelerated, the enzymes will become active, and the blood will not be suitable for human transfusion. If the temperature is too low, the nutrients will not be utilized, and there is a limited additional danger of accidental freezing, which will cause the cells to rupture.

Immediately before blood is issued for transfusion to a patient it should be carefully inspected by a technologist and the results of the inspection recorded. An important point to look for is evidence of hemolysis or any alteration in the color of the plasma. This could be indicative of excess red cell destruction or bacterial contamination with cryophilic organisms. Either of these conditions could lead to severe reactions in the recipient; blood suspected of being in this condition should not be issued.

BLOOD COMPONENT THERAPY

Modern technological advances have made it possible to separate whole blood into its component parts in such a manner that each can be used for its own beneficial effects. Thus it is possible to prepare red cells for the treatment of anemia, platelets for bleeding disorders, granulocytes for treatment of infection, and plasma factors for hemophilia from a single unit of blood. This permits not only a more efficient use of whole blood but also a far superior therapeutic regimen.[1]

The components of whole blood normally prepared in the modern blood bank along with some others made in sophisticated plasma fractionation plants are listed in Table 1. A number of acceptable methods can be used for the preparation of

TABLE 1. WHOLE BLOOD AND ITS COMPONENTS[8]

Component	Quantity	Shelf Life	Indications
Whole blood	450 ml blood 40% hematocrit	21–35 days @ 4C	Whole blood loss
Packed Red Cells	280 ml 70% hematocrit	See text	Anemia
Platelet concentrate	30–50 ml 5.5×10^{10}	72 hours @ 22C	Bleeding, platelet disorders
Granulocyte Concentrate	400 ml 2×10^{10}	< 24 hours @ 4C	Infections, granulocyte disorders
Fresh Frozen Plasma	225 ml 13 g protein	1 year @ −30C	Bleeding disorder, hypovolemia
Cryoprecipitate	10 ml 80 AHF units	1 year @ −30C	Hemophilia
Factor VIII Concentrate	1,000 units	2 years @ 2–8C	Hemophilia
Albumin 5%/25%	250–500 ml/ 50–100 ml	3 years @ 22C	Hypovolemia
Immune Serum Globulin	2–10 ml	3 years @ 2–8C	Hypogammaglobulinemia, Prophylaxis in virus infections

blood components. These will vary from one center to another depending on the equipment being used and the professional judgment of the director of the facility. Therefore, the methods described in this section are generalizations designed to illustrate the basic principles. For a more detailed description of the methodologies the reader is advised to consult other works and the standard operating procedure manual of the individual institution.[1, 2]

The most frequently used and most easily prepared component consists of packed red blood cells. These can be made simply by expressing the plasma from a unit of blood in which the red cells have been allowed to settle by gravity. However, a much more effective way of preparing this component is to centrifuge the unit of blood in a horizontal head refrigerated centrifuge for five minutes at 5,000 g. This will pack the red cells to the bottom of the bag, allow the leukocytes to settle on the surface, and leave the platelets in suspension in the plasma.

This type of treatment may change the expiration of the unit of blood. If the unit was originally collected into a double pack—two bags interconnected by tubing—the plasma can be expressed into the empty satellite bag without breaking the hermetic seal of the original unit. In such a case the expiration date of the packed cells is identical to that of the whole blood from which they were prepared. On the other hand, if the unit was collected into a single bag, the hermetic seal must be broken to attach an empty satellite bag for the plasma. Since the seal is broken, there is a layer of inadvertent bacterial contamination; therefore the packed cells made in this manner must be used within twenty-four hours of preparation. If they are not used within the allotted time, they must be discarded.

As a general rule, whenever components are prepared in a way that does not disturb the integrity of the original container, the dating period is identical to that of the whole blood. However, if the integrity must be broken for any reason the product is usable for only twenty-four hours.

Another component that is prepared frequently and with relative ease is platelet concentrate, either from a single donor or from up to ten individual donors. Platelets must be separated from whole blood immediately after collection. The blood is first centrifuged lightly at 1,740 g for about three minutes. This settles the red cells and white cells but allows the platelets to float free in the plasma. The platelet-rich plasma is expressed from the primary collection bag into an attached satellite pouch and the entire unit is recentrifuged at a higher relative centrifugal (5,000 g for five minutes) force. This sediments the platelets, allowing the clarified plasma to be returned to the red cells or removed for further chemical fractionation. Platelets prepared in this fashion have a shelf life of seventy-two hours. They must be maintained at room temperature and constantly agitated to prevent excessive aggregation.

Leukocytes for transfusion are usually prepared only in highly sophisticated donor centers. The quantity of these cells available for harvest from a single unit of whole blood is too small to be of any therapeutic value. Therefore, continuous flow methods must be used that allow multiple units of blood to be removed from the donor, the white cells extracted, and the remaining components returned to the donor's circulation. Under certain conditions drugs such as steroids or hydroxy ethyl starch are administered to the donor beforehand to increase the number of leukocytes in the circulating vascular pool. Because granulocytes are unstable, this component has a shelf life of less than twenty-four hours.

The plasma recovered as the result of the immediate preparation of packed cells may be frozen quickly and stored for up to one year at −30C as a source of Factor VIII and other coagulation factors. The cryoprecipitate formed after rapidly freezing the plasma and slowly thawing it at 4° C is an even richer source of Factor VIII. This can be removed and preserved, after which the remaining material can be fractionated into albumin and gamma globulin.

FROZEN BLOOD

The search to extend the storage of red blood cells indefinitely has been actively pursued since 1950.[3] At that time, it was found that erythrocytes could be freeze preserved, reconstituted with a minimum of hemolysis, and still retain their in vivo function.[4] According to the present-day state of the art, red blood cells, drawn into either CPD or CPD-Adenine anticoagulant solutions, remain usable for three years if stored frozen.

Units of donated erythrocytes are frozen and stored in the modern blood bank for a number of reasons other than just to extend their shelf life. Autologous red cells from patients with multiple alloantibodies can be stored for the patient's own use. In addition, cryopreserved cells can be used to provide an inventory of donors who possess rare blood groups and therefore are normally in short supply. Finally, such a repository of cells can be used to supplement the normal inventory when current blood donations are at a low ebb.

Unprotected erythrocytes separated from their plasma cannot be frozen without incurring a great deal of damage. These cells, just like all mammalian cells, contain water, which, when frozen, forms ice crystals. The length and size of these crystals depends on the freezing rate of the solution. Slow freezing rates usually result in the production of large ice crystals, whereas a very rapid rate of freezing produces smaller ones. It is known that cellular damage leading to membrane rupture is caused by this transformation of water into ice and the associated growth of crystals. However, it is unclear whether the ice crystals themselves disrupt the red cell membranes by physical displacement and shear effects; whether the damage results from a high salt concentration gradient that forms when the pure water crystallizes out of solution; or possibly a combination of the two. The major fact remains that when ice crystal formation is prevented, the cells' membranes remain intact.

One of the methods that can be used to prevent intracellular ice crystal formation is the addition of a penetrating cryoprotective agent. This is a type of substance that can readily diffuse into the cells and bind the water molecules in such a way that ice crystal formation cannot take place.

Currently, glycerol is the additive of choice for the freeze preservation of red blood cells. It is considered the best of the intracellular additives for human use because it allows only minimal structural damage during freezing and thawing, provided that procedures are carried out properly.

A solution of glycerol that also contains a nonpenetrating or extracellular cryoprotectant such as dextrose or fructose is superior to glycerol alone. Using both types of cryoprotective agents results in the formation of firm hydrogen bonds not only with the intracellular water trapped inside the cell but also with any water outside of the cell that is present in the residual plasma and anticoagulant solution. The combined reduction in the degree of ice crystal formation both inside and outside the cells results in a more effective reduction in damage. The glycerol-fructose solution is easily removed when the frozen red cell mass is reconstituted, and therefore is nontoxic to the potential recipient.

The key element of good freeze-preservation technique is to create conditions that will allow the cryoprotective agents to bind the water effectively and at the same time prevent the occurrence of excessive hypertonicity, which may result from the additive solution. Penetration of the glycerol is more rapid at temperatures higher than 4C. Therefore, the red cell mass and the glycerol solution should be combined at ambient temperature. Equilibration of the glycerol red cell mass should be achieved before the freezing process is begun. This allows for maximum hydrogen bonding between the glycerol and available water and minimizes the possibility of localized hypertonic conditions that could lead to excessive membrane shrinkage and rupture.

The freeze-preservation procedure may be carried out using two acceptable methods: 1. the slow freeze method of Huggins[5] using an 8.6 M solution of glycerol, or 2. the fast freeze method of Meryman[6] using a 4.6 M solution of glycerol. Blood frozen slowly is usually stored at −90C in mechanical freezers, whereas fast frozen blood is stored in vapor phase liquid nitrogen refrigerators at −193C.

Certain precautions must be observed in the maintenance of red cells in the frozen state. Blood preserved according to the Huggins method is stored in soft plastic bags, which become very brittle at the extremely low temperatures employed. Therefore care should be exercised when handling such units to avoid accidental cracking. Second, the mechanical refrigeration systems employed may break down during the storage period and must be monitored constantly.

Although metal containers are used in the Meryman technique, thereby avoiding the problems of breakage, the liquid nitrogen refrigerators are not failsafe. For example, the liquid nitrogen coolant in the storage chamber could be depleted if automatic filling does not occur due to a malfunction of appropriate electronic sensors or due to a failure to refill the reservoir tank at regular intervals. Therefore, regardless of the method, a repository of frozen blood cannot be left unattended.

The reconstitution techniques used to process the frozen red cell mass into a unit of transfusable red cells are probably more critical than the freezing procedures.[7] Again, the prevention of ice crystal growth during the thawing period is of paramount importance. This is accomplished by thawing the frozen red cells as rapidly as possible. In practice the container of frozen cells is removed from the freezer and immediately submerged into a water bath at 39C. The water in the bath should be agitated constantly to prevent it from cooling in the vicinity of the container and thus allowing crystal growth. The container must remain submerged until the contents are thawed completely. Once this has been accomplished the thawed red cell mass can be reconstituted.

Reconstitution is a process that involves the removal of the glycerol cryoprotective agent along with any other additives and restores the red cells to their normal physiologic condition. This may be accomplished either by a procedure known as agglomeration or by the use of a continuous-flow cell-washing centrifuge.

Agglomeration is a method of washing based on the principle that red cells clump and rapidly sediment when exposed to glucose solutions. The supernatant can be removed and the clumps uniformly dispersed by the addition of saline. The process may be repeated any number of times and avoids the use of a centrifuge.

In this method of reconstitution, a hypertonic, 12% glucose solution is added as the agglomerating agent. This is followed with four liters of 5% fructose to displace the intracellular glycerol. After decantation of the final wash solution, 0.85% saline is added to disperse the agglomerated red cells and restore physiologic conditions.

Deglycerolization with the continuous-flow cell washer is accomplished with a series of sodium chloride solutions of different concentrations. First a 12% solution is used to shrink the red cells, thereby forcing out the intracellular cryoprotectant. This is followed by a 1.6% solution to wash away the expressed glycerol. Finally, the red cells are returned to normal osmotic balance by washing with a 0.85% saline solution.

Regardless of the deglycerolization procedure used, the final saline wash is removed and the blood is issued for transfusion as packed cells. Because these procedures require multiple manipulations, freshly thawed blood has a shelf life of twenty-four hours.

The glycerol content of the red cells after successful reconstitution is less than 1% if the procedure is performed properly. However, a breach in technique can result in an increased rate of in vivo red cell destruction leading to possible hemoglobinemia and/or hemoglobinuria. This occurs because a greater than 1% residual intercellular glycerol concentration induces the rapid entry of water from plasma into the transfused red cells, causing them to swell and burst.

At the present time, routine cryopreservation is limited to red blood cells. However, studies indicate that the process can be used to store other elements, such as leukocytes and platelets. This will eliminate waste even further and help to satisfy the ever-increasing need for these components.

Review Questions

1. Describe the administrative operation of a blood bank.
2. Where does a blood bank obtain its blood?
3. What is the stigma associated with blood from paid donors?
4. What is provided by a department of hemotherapy other than blood and components for the patients it serves?

5. List five items that should be contained in a good laboratory procedure manual.
6. How should blood be inspected before it is released for transfusion?
7. Why is glycerol used in freezing red blood cells?
8. What is a disadvantage of using glycerol as a cryoprotective agent in freezing red cells?
9. Which blood component is given to patients with thrombocytopenia?
10. What is the choice of component for severe anemia?
11. What is the blood component best used for hemophiliacs?
12. What does autologous transfusion mean?

REFERENCES

1. Huestis DW, Bove JR, and Busch S: Practical Blood Transfusion. 3rd ed. Boston, Little, Brown, 1981.
2. American Association of Blood Banks: Technical Methods and Procedures. 7th ed. Washington, DC, AABB, 1977.
3. Smith Audrey A: Prevention of hemolysis during freezing and thawing of red cells. Lancet ii, 910, 1950.
4. Mollison PL and Sloviter HH: Successful transfusion of previously frozen human red cells. Lancet ii, 862, 1951.
5. Huggins CE: Frozen blood: Principles of practical preservation. Monographs in Surgical Sciences 3:133, 1966.
6. Meryman HT and Hornblower N: A method for freezing and washing red blood cells using a high glycerol concentration. Transfusion 12:145, 1966.
7. Valeri CR: Simplification of the methods for adding and removing glycerol during freeze-preservation of human red blood cells with high and low glycerol methods: biochemical modification prior to freezing. Transfusion 15:195, 1975.
8. Lee C Ling and Henry JB. In Todd Sanford Davidsohn: Clinical Diagnosis and Management by Laboratory Methods, Henry JB (ed), 16th ed. Philadelphia, W.B. Saunders, 1979, p 1468.

CHAPTER 3

Donor Room Techniques

Objectives

From the material presented in this chapter the student should be able to:

1. Gain an appreciation for the importance of personal interaction with blood donors.
2. Describe professional attitudes and their impact on nonmedical volunteers who come into a hospital setting.
3. Discuss the source and intended impact of the regulations governing blood donations on the donor and the recipient.
4. Conduct a medically useful donor interview.
5. Understand the rationale for the physical and laboratory examinations performed on donors.
6. Describe the basic principles of phlebotomy.
7. Understand the concept of pheresis and its mode of implementation.

Prospective blood donors, who are the sole source of a constant supply of blood and blood components for the blood bank, are very important people and should be accorded a cordial welcome by courteous and understanding blood bank personnel. The reception of the uninitiated blood donor is the origin of good public relations between the public and the hospital or community blood bank. The receptionist or secretary with whom the donor first comes in contact, as well as the technologists performing the phlebotomy, must be models of decorum and exhibit a professional attitude of behavior and appearance. In addition, these individuals should be knowledgeable and capable of developing a public understanding of the functions of the blood bank, of allaying the fear of the blood donation by explaining the methods employed and the medical reasons for blood replacement, and of describing the blood donor standards and how they protect both the donors and the prospective recipients.

A pleasant experience on initial exposure to blood donation can lead to the donors' eventual participation in the development of or the continuation of existing therapeutic platelet- and leukapheresis programs. Needless to say, such programs are wholly dependent on the good will of people who are willing to contribute time and be inconvenienced as well as undergoing some personal discomfort to provide these much needed cellular components.

RECEPTION, DONOR EXAMINATION, BLOOD COLLECTION, AND PHERESIS SPACES

The planning of the reception and donor examination rooms as well as the blood collection and pheresis spaces is one of the most important functions in designing the physical layout of the blood bank. Foreseeing peak loads and making provisions to care for them is paramount.

The objectives include the steady and orderly flow of donors through the efficient use of the blood bank personnel and equipment, thereby expediting the blood donations and preparation of pheresis products. In this manner, an atmosphere is created in which the work can be completed in as short a time as possible without causing the donor to experience any adverse physical or emotional reactions.

When possible, the reception, donor examination, blood collection, and pheresing spaces should adjoin one another, but they should not be located close to the working areas of the blood bank laboratory. Segregating these spaces from the working areas will prevent or minimize unnecessary personnel traffic and maintain low noise levels.

Reception Room

Careful attention should be given to the planning of reception space. The room should be large enough to accommodate the anticipated peak load of donors. It should be attractively decorated, well lighted and ventilated, with monitored temperature. Comfortable furnishings should be provided, including an adequate number of chairs, tables, and racks for magazines, as well as clothes racks and umbrella stands. To add to the donors' comfort, rest rooms should be located next to the reception space and a public telephone should be nearby.

Donors in hospital centers often come to replace the blood that was administered to one of their relatives or friends; therefore, the secretary-receptionist should be provided with an up-to-date list of the transfusions given to patients and previous blood donations credited to those patients' accounts. This should be done for purposes of record keeping. Monetary discussions should be referred to the business office handling the patients' accounts.

In practice, the receptionist registers the prospective donors, searches the files for evidence of previous donations, and fills in the donor record cards with the date of the current donation, the donor's name and source of positive identification, address, age, sex, patient to be credited with the donation, and the place and date of last blood donation.

Donor Qualifications

The Bureau of Biologics (BOB) has codified the acceptable qualifications of people who may be allowed to donate blood and blood components. The regulations are designed to protect the donors themselves, the patients who receive the product, and the institutions that draw the blood and produce the blood components. The regulations are minimal and may be superceded by stringent state or local regulations. In some extenuating circumstances deemed in the best medical interest of the donor any of these regulations may be modified by a qualified physician. Thus the department of hemotherapy must be knowledgeable about the local, state, and federal regulations concerning the operation of a donor facility.

Briefly, a person must be deemed acceptable to donate whole blood or blood components by a qualified physician, or by people trained to determine the suitability of a donor and who are supervised by a qualified physician. Each prospective donor must have a medical history, a test for hemoglobin level, and a physical examination as prescribed by the medical director of the blood bank. A manual of standard procedures may be used when the physician is not present on the premises.

Age. Donors are acceptable between the ages of seventeen through sixty-five. Donors who do not meet these requirements may donate with the written consent of their parents or guardian if they are under seventeen, or the approval of a blood bank physician if they are over sixty-six.

Donors engaged in hazardous occupations cannot be considered for donation unless it can be established that suitable time for recovery from the donation is available. The appropriate recovery time between the blood donation and the resumption of the hazardous occupation is generally twenty-four hours, the only exception being an extension of the recovery period to seventy-two hours for flight crews.

Medical Examination

The medical examination is the most important part of the predonation workup. It is designed to ensure the safety of the donor by uncovering underlying medical problems that could lead to excessive discomfort or sudden and unexpected harm from the loss of a unit of whole blood. It is also meant to safeguard the potential recipient from any undesirable effects, such as infection with bacterial, fungal, viral, or parasitic agents, accidental introduction of unwanted drugs or metabolic wastes, or poor therapeutic effect resulting from the blood of a generally unhealthy donor.

The examination consists of two parts, a concise history pertinent to the donation and a brief physical examination. The history must be taken at the time of each donation regardless of the number of previous times the person donated blood. It should be conducted in privacy, and strict confidentiality must be maintained at all times. A portion of the physical examination consists of taking the donor's oral temperature. The interviewer is cautioned to postpone this event until the conclusion of the interview, since it is extremely difficult and potentially dangerous to answer questions with a thermometer in one's mouth.

Donor History

Most donor centers have a donor card listing the pertinent questions to be asked during the taking of the history. However, the donor should not be allowed to complete this form. Rather, the person taking the history should ask each question clearly and distinctly. The interviewer should note not only the response given but should also observe the donor and his or her reaction to the particular question. This is important because some donors, in their zeal to donate or because of personal embarrassment, may be less than totally truthful about their responses, a situation that could lead to potentially serious consequences. Anything other than negative responses to any of the medical questions is considered immediate grounds for the rejection of the donor. Typically the donor is queried about the following:

Date of last donation. Donations are allowed every eight weeks, but not more often than four times per calendar year.

Previous rejection as a donor. The circumstances surrounding the previous rejection must be elucidated to determine whether they still prevail. If the condition has been corrected the donor may be accepted; however, persistence of an undesirable attribute may preclude further consideration.

Viral hepatitis. A history of a viral hepatitis infection is a cause for permanent rejection of a donor. This is extended to include a reactive HB$_s$Ag test, or being the sole donor of a unit of blood or a component received by a recipient who developed posttransfusion hepatitis. To further safeguard against the possible transmission of hepatitis, people who may have been accidentally infected are rejected temporarily for at least six months. This would include donors who have been in close contact with a person who had a viral hepatitis infection and donors who themselves have received whole blood or blood components within the past six months.

People who have had tattoos, earpiercing, skin allografts, and acupuncture are also rejected for six months. Finally, any donor who was one of a group of donors transfused into a patient who later developed posttransfusion hepatitis should be evaluated by the blood bank physician regarding suitability as a blood donor.

Malaria. Donors who have traveled in an endemic malarial zone within the past six months are rejected until the six-month quarantine has expired. Donors who have lived in an endemic malarial zone are rejected for a period of three years. World charts of malarial zones are available to blood banks from the Malarial Program, Center for Disease Control, U.S. Public Health Service, and from the American Association of Blood Banks. Donors who have had malarial attacks or antimalarial prophylaxis within three years of a blood donation are also rejected.

Syphilis. People presenting a history of current or past syphilis are rejected. Written proof of having received adequate therapy and a return to the seronegative condition may be acceptable when the donor is examined by the blood bank physician.

Pregnancy. Pregnancy or delivery within the past six weeks are grounds for rejection. Exceptions to this rule are made in the case of an autologous blood donor who may be donating for her own use, for the treatment of hemolytic disease due to unusual red cell alloantibodies in her own child, or for the procurement of material platelets for the treatment of neonatal thrombocytopenia.

Abnormal bleeding tendencies. Donors with histories of hemophilia, purpura, homoptysis, and bleeding ulcers are rejected for their own protection. For the same reason donors may be temporarily rejected if they have a history of hemorrhoids or immediate postmenstrual bleeding.

Convulsions or fainting spells. A history of convulsions or fainting spells after the age of three are an indication of some permanent neurological disorder and constitute a cause for rejection on the grounds of donor protection.

Minor surgery and tooth extraction. Prospective donors who have had tooth extractions are excluded from donating for seventy-two hours, since such procedures invite bacterial infections that will not become evident until a suitable period of incubation is allowed to elapse.

Other items. All donors are questioned as to their general state of health. Obviously, diseases of the heart, kidney, or liver, in addition to a history of prior malignancy, are grounds for exclusion. Previous active immunization with bacterial or viral antigens may require postponement of donation depending on materials used. The same is true for a history of tuberculosis. Careful inquiry as to the use of any medications, no matter how trivial it may seem to the donor, should be made. Inadvertently a donor may not mention a drug that could clearly be grounds for rejection. For example, even the use of aspirin would be cause for concern in a donor being platelet pheresed. The blood bank physician should be consulted in such cases.

In addition, the interviewer should inspect the donor to ascertain that he or she looks healthy and shows no evidence of being under the influence of alcohol or drugs. Finally, the interviewer should inspect both arms for any signs of narcotics addiction.

TABLE 1. ACCEPTABLE VALUES FOR DONORS

Determination	Acceptable Value
Hemoglobin	Female: 12.5 g/dl Male: 13.5 g/dl
Hematocrit	Female: 38% Male: 41%
Pulse	50–100
Blood Pressure	Diastolic: 50–100 mm Hg Systolic: 90–180 mm Hg
Weight	110 lbs (50 kg)*

* 50 kg is the minimum weight at which a full unit of 450 ± 45 ml along with up to 30 ml of blood for pilot samples can be collected. Proportionately less blood with correspondingly less anticoagulant must be collected if the donor does not meet this minimum weight. Under no circumstances can more than the allotted total volume of blood be removed regardless of weight without a physician's specific approval.

Physical examination. The physical examination is conducted to ascertain that the donor is physically able to lose a unit of blood. Tests are done to obtain an estimate of the blood volume and total red cell mass, and blood pressure and heart rate are determined. The oral temperature should be taken at this time and must be no higher than 37.5C. Normal values for these determinations are given in Table 1. Any abnormalities should not be discussed with the donor without first consulting with the blood bank physician.

Required Laboratory Tests. Certain serologic tests must be performed on the serum of the donor at the time of each donation of either a single unit of blood or a pheresis component. The first of these is a test to rule out the presence of syphilis, which could infect a potential recipient. The RPR is normally performed to satisfy this requirement, and anyone found to be positive cannot be used as a donor.

There is some question as to the real value of this procedure in protecting the intended recipient. First, most serologic tests for syphilis are nonspecific indicators of the presence of an antibody to *Treponema pallidum*, the organism in question. Second, the only donors who are capable of transmitting the disease are those with an active spirochetemia. However, in that particular stage of the disease, the serologic tests are most frequently negative. Despite these drawbacks, the test is still mandatory as of this writing, although there are movements to have this requirement rescinded.

The second mandatory test is a "third generation" test for the presence of the hepatitis B surface antigen (HB_sAg). Third generation is a category referring to the degree of sophistication and sensitivity of the test procedure and it includes radioimmunoassay and passive hemagglutination inhibition assays, which are the latest ones developed. This test has been shown to be particularly valuable in reducing the incidence of posttransfusion hepatitis infection. People found to be positive for the presence of the HB_sAg antigen are considered potentially infectious and cannot be used as donors. However, it must be pointed out that the procedure as currently employed is capable of identifying only the Type B hepatitis virus carrier. There is another form of hepatitis that is caused by a Type A virus and still another that is neither Type A nor Type B (the so-called non-A, non-B). Tests are currently being developed to detect Type A, but no practical method is yet in sight to detect non-A, non-B. Therefore, it should be borne in mind that even though all donors can be identified as presumably noninfectious with respect to one type of hepatitis virus, a certain risk of the disease still remains.

THE PHLEBOTOMY

The term *phlebotomy* is used to describe the procedure of piercing the vein with an instrument for the purpose of collecting blood. When it is carried out to obtain blood for transfusion, a relatively large needle must be used to ensure a good flow and to prevent clotting. As a result the technologist should consider it a minor surgical procedure and perform it accordingly.

Although little risk is involved, certain precautions must be taken to guard against infecting either the donor or the blood being collected. One of the simplest rules, but one that is most often forgotten, is that the operator must wash his or her hands before each phlebotomy and before attending to another donor. Technologists' hands, especially in a hospital, are a rich source of pathogenic bacteria that can easily contaminate either the donor or the instruments being used. Furthermore, in preparing a donor for phlebotomy one must push up the sleeve, palpate the vein, apply the tourniquet, and in other ways pick up organisms on the donor's skin. Unless the hands are washed before attending the next donor, the possibility of cross-contamination exists.

The donor's skin must be thoroughly disinfected before the needle is inserted. Obviously the skin is the home of a multitude of microbes. During the course of the phlebotomy a small plug of skin is cut out, which is normally flushed into the blood container. Unless the skin has been rendered as bacteria-free as possible, the organisms present can infect the blood. Furthermore, bacteria adjacent to skin puncture can be swept along the needle track directly into the donor's vein. This can result in the potential development of phlebitis.

Under normal circumstances it is impossible to render the donor's skin sterile. However, it is possible to achieve a state of surgical cleanliness. This is accomplished with successive scrubs to remove excess dirt and natural skin oils, followed by a germicide containing iodine, and finally a solvent to remove excess iodine that may cause irritation.

A generous area of the antecubital space of the forearm should be scrubbed (about three to four inches in diameter) in the vicinity of the venipuncture. The swabbing sponges currently used are sterile, already impregnated with the appropriate solution, and individually packaged ready for use. They must not be handled with the fingers but rather with hemostats reserved for that purpose and kept in a container of germicide solution.

Contrary to popular belief, scrubbing the skin in the surgical sense is not scrubbing at all. The swab should be gently but firmly rubbed over the skin in a series of concentric circles, beginning over the intended site of venipuncture and progressing to the outermost surface. Once a swab is moved to the outside it should never be returned to the center. When the scrub is complete, the area is covered with a sterile gauze compress to protect it from the air. The scrubbing should be performed only after the intended vein is distended by the application of a suitable tourniquet (a blood pressure cuff inflated to about 50 mm Hg is most comfortable and normally used) and the area palpated. Once the scrub is complete, the operator's fingers must not touch the area of puncture until the needle has been inserted.

Blood containers come with an integral donor tube to which is affixed a sterile needle covered with a sheath. To preserve this sterility, care should be taken to remove the sheath immediately before use so that the needle will not be touched and thereby contaminated. If the vein is missed and the blood fails to flow, another site must be scrubbed and a new blood collection set must be employed.

During collection, the donor should be watched to observe any untoward reaction and the blood bag agitated by squeezing to ensure adequate mixing with the anticoagulant. When a sufficient amount of blood has been collected, as evidenced by the weight of the bag, the donor tube is clamped off, the tourniquet loosened, and the needle removed. At the same time pressure is applied to the puncture site and the donor should be asked to elevate the arm until the blood ceases to ooze.

In the meantime, the blood in the donor tube is stripped into the bag, mixed with anticoagulant, and then allowed to refill the tubing. The tubing can then be sealed off into appropriate segments.

SPECIAL CONSIDERATIONS FOR PHERESIS

It is now routine practice to prepare large quantities of certain blood components, namely plasma, platelets, and leukocytes, by pheresis procedures. This is a technique in which whole blood is withdrawn from a donor, the desired component separated, and the unneeded elements such as red cells returned to the donor.

The procedure has two major advantages. The first is that a large volume of the component can be obtained from a single donor, more than that normally found in a single unit of blood. Second, the same donor may be called on at more frequent intervals than those specified for the donation of whole blood, provided that a unit of blood is not lost in the process.

This procedure can be carried out in its simplest form by drawing a unit of blood from a donor through a special collection set that has two parts connected by a "Y" adapter. The collection bag is connected to one area of the "Y" and a bottle of sterile normal saline to the other. The blood is drawn into the bag and the passage into the veins is kept open with a slow saline drip, while the component is prepared. When this is completed, the bag containing the remaining red cells is reconnected and the cells are reinfused after being resuspended in some of the sterile saline.

The method, although useful, is cumbersome and has certain disadvantages. It takes a long time, is not very efficient, and suffers from the dangers of clerical errors if more than one donor at a time is being pheresed. Furthermore, if the bag of blood being processed is damaged, the red cells can not be reinfused and the donor is lost for eight weeks.

Newer methods of pheresis employ continuous-flow instruments such as those illustrated in Chapter 1. These machines are basically a centrifuge with a specially designed continuous-flow bowl with several ports through which materials can flow in and out. The bowls are disposable, come presterilized, and are made to hold about one unit of blood. The phlebotomy needle is inserted into a vein in one of the donor's arms and the blood is allowed to flow into the bowl, where it is mixed with ACD solution as an anticoagulant. The bowl is spun, and, because of its design, the red cells, white cells, platelets, and plasma are separated. A series of cleverly designed valves makes it possible to divert the flow of each of these elements into separate pouches. The pouches containing the desired components are clamped off and the remaining material is pumped into a reservoir from which it is reinfused into a second vein in the donor's other arm. The process is continuous, so that fresh blood keeps refilling the spinning bowl as the components are removed. Using this method, one can collect large amounts of certain components, such as platelets, in a relatively short period of time without any appreciable alteration in the donor's red cell mass.

Pheresis is an invasive procedure and must be performed under the strict supervision of the blood bank physician. A number of precautions must be taken to safeguard the donor. First, stringent aseptic conditions must be maintained throughout. Since more equipment is handled and two venipunctures are employed, at least twice the chance of infection is present. Second, during the procedure the calcium-binding anticoagulant ACD is used to prevent clotting and is eventually injected into the donor via the reinfused red cells. Therefore, there is the attendant danger of hypocalcemia, requiring careful monitoring of the donor. Third, the donor blood is subjected to some degree of trauma from the centrifugation and the action of the various pumps and valves. As a result, some of the red cells could be damaged and free hemoglobin released into the suspending fluid. A close check must be made on the material being reinfused for the presence of this protein. Fourth, if the product being removed is plasma there is the danger of hypovolemia, so the donor's fluid balance must be monitored. Finally, donors who are subjected to this procedure routinely must be evaluated to ensure that their supply of whatever product is being harvested is not overly depleted. This may entail periodic white counts, platelet counts, and/or serum protein levels, along with electrophoresis and the quantitation of immunoglobulin levels.

Review Questions

1. What are the proper steps (in their appropriate sequence) for preparing the phlebotomy site before donation of blood?
2. What periodic determinations are required in quality control of platelet preparations?
3. What should you do if, on routine screening, a donor sample is found to be HB$_s$Ag positive?
4. What disease is transmissable to a recipient by transfusion of plasma?
5. What is the maximum blood pressure of a donor?
6. On what does the expiration date of blood components depend?
7. How often may a person in good health donate blood?
8. How are platelets separated from whole blood?
9. Why are donors who have received blood or blood products within six months of the time of donation rejected?
10. List three reasons for rejecting donors for their own protection.
11. Give two instances in which donors are rejected to protect the recipient.

REFERENCES

1. American Association of Blood Banks: Standards for Blood Banks and Transfusion Services. 10th ed. Washington, DC, AABB, 1981.
2. Code of Federal Regulation Title 21. Food and Drugs. Washington, DC, US Government Printing Office, 1980.
3. Huestis DW, Bove JR, and Busch S: Practical Blood Transfusion. 3rd ed. Boston, Little, Brown, 1981.

CHAPTER 4

Serologic Methods Used in Blood Grouping

Objectives

The information presented in this chapter should enable the student to:

1. Describe the general properties of antigens.
2. Explain the biological mechanism and cellular dynamics of the immune response.
3. Understand the structural and functional properties of antibodies and the concept of antibody heterogeneity.
4. Describe the concept of serologic specificity.
5. Understand the basic nature of serologic reactions and the way in which they can be manipulated by altering the physicochemical environment.
6. Learn the difference between complete and incomplete antibodies.
7. Understand the features of the direct and the indirect antiglobulin test.
8. Develop an appreciation for the properties and functions of the complement system.
9. Learn to use commonly available blood grouping reagents intelligently.

Karl Landsteiner (Fig. 1) was the first to point out that there are immunologic differences among the red blood cells of various people.[1] These differences, referred to as human blood groups, are a series of genetically controlled polymorphic antigenic determinants that can be detected by means of their interaction with specific antibodies.

Blood group antigens are relatively easy to define in the modern laboratory using simple serologic procedures and readily available reagents. However, this aspect of the service load constitutes only a part of the laboratory's function. The remainder consists of preparing and ascertaining that a particular unit of blood can be transfused into a given patient with no harmful effects. Since most such harmful effects result from blood group antigen-antibody interactions, a basic understanding of some of the immunologic principles governing in vivo antibody production and behavior as well as in vitro antibody reactivity is an essential prerequisite for any prospective worker in the blood bank laboratory.

ANTIGENS

In the broadest sense, an antigen can be any substance that has the ability to evoke an in vivo immune response upon parenteral injection into an immunologically competent animal. In addition, it can react with the products of such a response either in vivo or in vitro.

One of the essential prerequisites for a material to be antigenic is that it be foreign to the host. Therefore, it must have a chemical configuration that is not normally present in the body of the responding animal or, if present, has been physi-

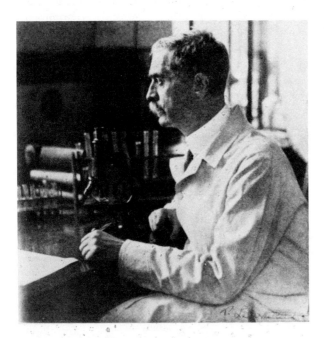

Fig. 1. Karl Landsteiner—Nobel laureate, the discoverer of the human blood groups and the founder of immunohematology. (*Courtesy of Trent Collection, Duke University Medical Center Library.*)

cally shielded from exposure to the immune system because of its anatomic location.

Under normal conditions the body has a built-in self-recognition mechanism, which prevents it from eliciting an immune response directed against itself. However, under certain pathologic conditions this built-in safety factor of the immunologic mechanism can be overcome or may break down and an immune response may be elicited by one's own body components. Such a series of events can lead to the production of an abnormal autoimmune disease.

It should be stressed, however, that autoimmunity is an unusual event. A much clearer understanding of the various concepts pertaining to the human blood groups and transfusion practice can be obtained if the concept that the immune response is evoked only by immunologically foreign materials and only in immunologically susceptible individuals is accepted as the normal situation.

The human blood group antigens identify differences among groups of humans that are a natural expression of polymorphic variation. Antigens that comprise very fine immunologic characteristics of a particular individual or of a group of individuals within the same species are called *alloantigens*. Alloantigens, because they define such fine differences among individuals of the same species, are not powerful immunogens. Even the strongest human blood group antigens are relatively weak in their general ability to provoke an immune response in other humans as compared to, for example, bacterial antigens. Nevertheless, under appropriate circumstances even very minute doses of red blood cells carrying such antigens can result in the production of a measurable antibody response.

In spite of their relatively poor immunogenic qualities, however, the blood groups of red cells can present substantial clinical problems in transfusion practice since most people, as will be discussed later, already possess certain preformed products of an immune response to some of the most important antigens. In addition, pregnancy and the extensive use of transfusion therapy furnish adequate amounts of antigenic material to make even the poorest antigens highly significant in clinical situations.

Blood group antigens, like all other antigenic materials, are large organic molecules having a rigid chemical structure composed of either proteins or large and often complex polysaccharides. Some antigens are made up of combinations of these chemical moieties that may on occasion contain lipids. This is especially true of cell membrane antigens.[2] Frequently, large proteins or lipid carriers may contribute the necessary size and cellular attachment, whereas polysaccharide or polypeptide structures, present in the form of side chains, confer the immunologic specificity. The side chains can be considered as ligands; that is, the antigenic determinant groups or combining sites with which the products of the immune response react.

THE IMMUNE RESPONSE

When an appropriate antigen or immunogen challenges the body, two types of immune responses can be elicited. The first results in the production of highly specific protein molecules, called antibodies, that ultimately appear in the serum of the immunized person. This event is called a *humoral immune response* and is the one with which we are primarily concerned when dealing with antigens of the formed elements of human blood. The second response that can be elicited is manifested by the production of antigen-specific immunologically committed killer cells. This form of response results in a condition known as *cellular immunity* or *delayed hypersensitivity* and is exemplified by the tuberculin reaction and the rejection of allografts (organ or tissue transplants).

The maintenance of a system of immunologic responsiveness is one of the major functions of the cells of the lymphoid tissue. The responsible element is made up of at least two distinct populations of small lymphocytes called T-cells and B-cells. Although morphologically identical, these two subpopulations of lymphocytes can be distinguished by certain detectable membrane markers. The most striking feature of T-cells is that they possess a receptor for sheep red blood cells. This allows sheep red cells to adhere to their surface when appropriately mixed in vitro. B-cells, on the other hand, carry immunoglobulins on their surface and on occasion within their cytoplasm.

The T-cells constitute about 60–80% of the total circulating peripheral blood lymphocytes and are those small lymphocytes that, having originated from bone marrow stem cells, are processed and brought to maturity by the thymus gland. This cell type is ultimately responsible for all aspects of cellular immunity. The B-cells, constituting an additional 20–25% of peripheral blood lymphocytes, originate in the bone marrow stem cells just like T-cells. However, they do not undergo thymic modification. Under the appropriate conditions resulting from antigenic challenge and with the assistance of T-cell helpers, they transform into plasma cells whose only function is humoral antibody production. A serum from an immunized person containing a collection of antibodies resulting from a specific immune response is called an antiserum.

The kind of immune response obtained, cellular or humoral, depends on the type of antigen used for its induction. It is believed that complicated antigens such as virus-infected cells are preferentially handled through a cellular response, whereas relatively simple antigens such as those expressed on the surface of red blood cells, with only a single or at most only a few antigenic determinants per molecule, induce a humoral response.

One of the most important characteristics of the immune response is the exquisite specificity of it and its products. This specificity can be demonstrated both in vivo and in vitro by numerous serologic reactions. One of Landsteiner's experiments[3] conducted many years ago and shown in Table 1 is a classic example of the degree of this specificity. In this experiment three optically isomeric haptens, *l*-tartaric, *d*-tartaric, and *m*-tartaric acids, which differ only in the juxtaposition of a hydrogen and hydroxyl group on the two central carbon atoms, were coupled to a carrier protein and used to immunize animals. The resultant antisera were capable of distinguishing these three isomeric compounds in serologic tests. From this result, it is possible to conclude that the antigenic determinant that is responsible for the specificity of the serologic reaction need be only a very small part of the larger immunogen.

A response such as this is not an all-or-nothing phenomenon. Purely qualitative differences may not be observed and the products can be distinguished only by

TABLE 1. THE REACTIVITY OF SERA PREPARED AGAINST THE ISOMERS OF TARTARIC ACID*

Antisera	Haptens		
	l-tartaric acid	*d*-tartaric acid	*m*-tartaric acid
	COOH	COOH	COOH
	|	|	|
	HOCH	HCOH	HCOH
	|	|	|
	HCOH	HOCH	HCOH
	|	|	|
	COOH	COOH	COOH
Anti-levo-tartaric acid	+++	±	±
Anti-dextro-tartaric acid	O	+++	±
Anti-meso-tartaric acid	±	O	+++

* After Landsteiner[3]

precise quantitative serologic techniques. For example, the antiserum produced in response to the dextrorotatory isomer reacts more strongly with it than with the levorotatory isomer, indicating that its major antibody component is anti-*d*-tartaric acid. The minor reactions observed with the l-form can be attributed to what is known as cross-reactivity. This results from the fact that the antiserum also contains a small number of antibodies that were produced whose specificity was directed against components of the molecule shared by the two isomeric forms. Usually the immune response is at first very selective in recognizing minute differences in antigenic molecules. Under continued exposure, however, this selectivity breaks down, and larger portions of the molecule begin to influence the response. The development of cross-reactive antibodies is a common occurrence even with natural antigens and in no way jeopardizes the concept of the specificity of immunologic reactions, since this concept refers to the specificity of a single antibody molecule for its particular antigenic determinant. The fact remains that there are a finite number of biochemical configurations that are compatible with life. It is not unreasonable to assume that a large number of these will be shared by various plants and animals both within and among species.

The antigenic determinant or *ligand* (that which attaches to an antibody) is frequently referred to as a *hapten.* This term, apart from its chemical usage, has another important immunologic definition. If one considers that an antigen is defined as a substance that can induce an immune response in vivo, and reacts with the products of this response in vitro, one can define a hapten as being a compound that cannot, by itself, provoke an immune response in vivo but can react with the products of that immune response in vitro. The pneumococcal type-specific polysaccharides are typical haptens. The injection of a polysaccharide purified from a single strain of bacterial organisms into rabbits or horses does not result in an active immune response. To obtain antibodies reactive with this substance, intact pneumococci must be injected. Nevertheless, once the antibodies are produced they will react specifically with the purified bacterial product. Whether or not any substance behaves as a hapten or as a full antigen depends to a large extent on the presence of specific gametic information in the species of animal being immunized. For, although the pneumococcal polysaccharides are haptenic when injected into rabbits or horses, they are fully antigenic and capable of eliciting a normal immune response in humans and mice.

CHARACTERISTICS OF ANTIBODIES

Antibodies are defined as specific serum proteins produced by the plasma cells in the lymphoid tissue as a result of stimulation with an antigen. Antibodies are capable of chemical union both in vivo and in vitro with the particular antigen responsible for their production. When the serum proteins are separated electrophoretically, antibody activity can be shown to be associated with those fractions found in the gamma globulin region composed of a heterogeneous population of molecules (Fig. 2). Other techniques, such as ultracentrifugal analysis, diffusion, and immunoelectrophoresis, which take into account not only the electrophoretic mobility but also the size, shape, and antigenic structure of the molecules, have demonstrated that there are many different forms of antibody globulin. These various forms have been grouped together under the general term *immunoglobulins* and are referred to as Ig. At present five distinct immunoglobulin classes been described in humans: IgM, IgG, IgA, IgD, and IgE. Some of the properties of these immunoglobulin isotypes are given in Table 2. Studies performed to date indicate that the majority of

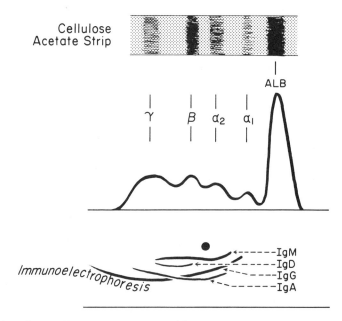

Fig. 2. The electrophoretic separation of human serum proteins on a cellulose acetate matrix is indicative of their heterogeneity. Notice the array of antigenically different immunoglobulins found in the area of the gamma region when the same serum is examined by immunoelectrophoresis.

TABLE 2. SOME PROPERTIES OF THE IMMUNOGLOBULINS FOUND IN HUMAN SERUM

Present Name	Previous Terms	Molecular Weight	Sedi-mentation Constant	Antibody Activity	Iso-Agglutinin Activity	Serum Concentration (mg/ml)	Principal Electro-phoretic Mobility
IgM	γ1M, β2M, 19Sγ, γMacro-globulin γM	900,000	18S (19S)	Yes	Complete	0.95–1.5	Between γ and β
IgG	γ, 7Sγ, 6.6Sγ, γ2 γss, γG	150,000	6.6S (7S)	Yes	Complete and incomplete	12–14	γ
IgA	β2A, γ1A γA	165,000	(9,11,13S) 6.6S	Yes	Incomplete, usually	2–4	Between γ and β
IgD	γ1S	150,000	7S	Some	?	0.003–0.03	Between γ and β
IgE		150,000	8S	Yes (reaginic)	?	0.0001–0.0006	?

37

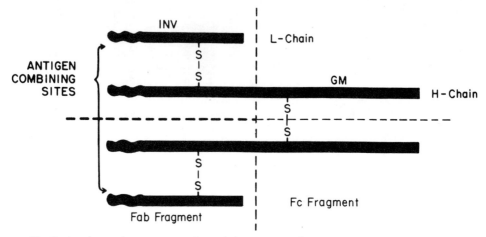

Fig. 3. A schematic representation of the structural components of the IgG molecule, which is a prototype of the basic monomeric configuration of all immunoglobulins. Enzymatic cleavage can be accomplished along the planes illustrated with dashed lines.

blood group antibodies are associated primarily with the IgM and IgG classes, although some belonging to the IgA classes do occur.

The 7S, or 150,000 Dalton, IgG immunoglobulin molecule has been studied extensively. Functionally it is a bivalent antibody with two sites available for combination with antigens. Chemical analyses of the products of enzymatic splitting of the molecules have revealed that it is composed of four chains, two light chains and two heavy chains held together by disulfide bridges. A diagrammatic representation of this molecule is shown in Figure 3.

Amino acid sequencing studies have shown that there are certain areas of in-

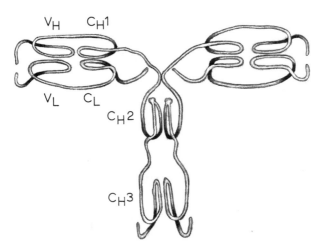

Fig. 4. A model of an immunoglobulin molecule, based on amino acid sequence studies, showing the loops created by intrachain disulfide bridges, which constitute the various functional domains. (*After Edelman.*[4])

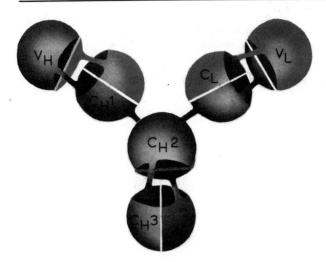

Fig. 5. An artist's conception of the three-dimensional structure with pivoting hinge regions (between C_H^1 and C_H^2), based on X-ray defraction studies of crystalline IgG. V_L and V_H are the domains composed of the regions of variable homology responsible for antigen recognition. C_L, C_H^1, C_H^2, and C_H^3 are the domains composed of the regions of constant homology responsible for effector function such as complement activation. (*After Poljak.*[5])

terchain homology with respect to the regular occurrence of certain amino acids within the IgG heavy chain and between portions of the heavy and light chains.[4] Each area of homology consists of approximately 110 amino acid residues, with about sixty of them making up a loop stabilized by intrachain disulfide bridges. A model of such a structure is shown in Figure 4.

Some of these are regions of homology referred to as V regions (two per molecule) and are composed of a variable portion of the terminal ends of the light and heavy chains. In addition, there are three other regions or *domains* that are constant in all IgG molecules of a particular individual regardless of the antibody specificity. One of the regions, C_L-C_H^1 (two per molecule), is composed of the remaining portion of the light chains and a segment of the heavy chains. The remaining two regions, C_H^2-C_H and C_H^3-C_H^3 (one each per molecule), include the rest of the length of the heavy chains. A three-dimensional representation of this molecular unit deduced from X-ray crystallography is shown in Figure 5.[5]

Studies on the other immunoglobulin classes have shown that their basic structure likewise consists of a pair of light and a pair of heavy chains having regions of homology similar to those found in IgG, except that IgM and IgE have five domains rather than four.

The actual antigen combining site, or the business end of the antibody, is contained within the variable domains of the light and heavy chains. The specificity of the antibody for its antigen is determined by a unique amino acid sequence, called a *hypervariable region,* within the variable domain.

The constant domains are responsible for investing the molecule with the particular attributes of its own immunoglobulin class. These include such characteristics as immunologically defined class and allospecificity as well as sites for complement activation, secretion, and placenta permeability.[6]

Various immunochemical and serologic studies have shown that the immunoglobulins have the shapes in Figure 6. A structure similar to that of IgG, having dimensions of 12.5 nm × 11.7 nm, forms a basic unit. The elegant electron micro-

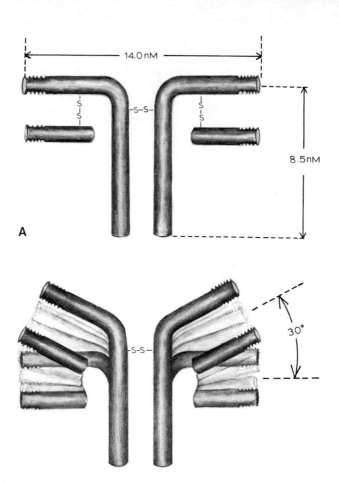

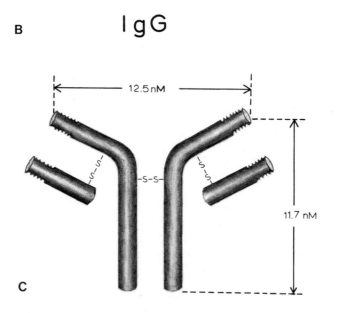

IgG

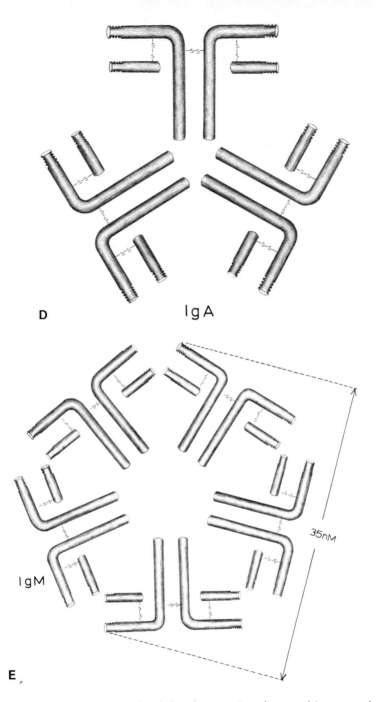

D

IgA

35nM

IgM

E

Fig. 6. A diagrammatic sketch of the three major classes of immunoglobulins and their relative sizes. **A.** IgG is a monomer of the basic unit. It is found in a "T" configuration in the native state. **B.** The arms carrying the light chains can swing through a thirty-degree arc in any direction at the hinge region, and **C.** upon combination with the antigen achieve and retain a "Y" configuration. **E.** IgM normally occurs as a pentamer of the basic unit while IgA is a trimer **D.** The threaded portion of each chain represents the variable region composed of a distinctive structure that allows for specific binding to the antigen. Unique amino acid sequencing in the heavy chain of each of the immunoglobulin classes allows immunologic differentiation in the various isotypes, G, M, A, E, and D.

graphs of Svehag[7] indicate that IgM is a pentamer of this unit with an effective length of 35 nm, while IgA may exist as single units, dimers, and trimers.

The study of Bence-Jones proteins, which are basically free light chains, has revealed that the L chains of all immunoglobulins (IgG, IgM, IgA, IgD, and IgE) are the same and may be one of two basic types, either κ or λ. The difference between κ and λ chains lies in their individual amino acid sequence. This difference imparts to each type of chain a characteristic antigenic property.

Whereas the light chains are shared by all immunoglobulin classes, the H chains are class specific and, therefore, different for each immunoglobulin type. Thus IgM has μ chains, IgG has γ chains, IgA has α chains, and so forth, each having distinct antigenic determinants. It is possible then to distinguish one immunoglobulin class from another on an immunologic basis using appropriately produced antisera.

Studies of human myeloma proteins, which consist of identical heavy chains produced by a single clone of cells, have shown that the chains of IgG can be further separated into four subclasses, each of which has unique antigenic groups. The antigenic differences among the four γ subclasses, γ G1, γ G2, γ G3, and γ G4, which affect their function and serologic properties as antibodies, are due to basic structural differences in the constant, C, regions of the heavy chains. Some of the properties of the IgG subclasses are summarized in Table 3.[8]

The gamma globulins, being serum proteins, carry certain amino acid sequences that are characteristic for their species of origin. However, antigenic differences in the gamma globulins among members of the same species also occur. These are referred to as *allotypes* and have been extensively studied in rabbits and humans.

The IgM immunoglobulin is much larger than IgG. Its sedimentation coefficient is 19S, with a molecular weight close to 1,000,000 Daltons, and it is often referred to as a macroglobulin.

Ordinarily, antibodies of the IgM class are formed early in the course of a primary immunization. Further stimulation with an antigen or a subsequent dose of an antigen results in a switchover to the production of antibodies of the IgG class.

TABLE 3. SOME PROPERTIES OF THE HUMAN γ HEAVY CHAIN SUBCLASSES

Subclasses	γ G1	γ G2	γ G3	γ G4
Percent total IgG	70	80	8	3
Gm factors	1,2,3,4,17,22	23	5,6,10,11,13 14,15,16,21	?
Interact with complement	Yes	Poorly	Yes	Not at all
Half life (days)	23	23	8	23
Antibody Activity	Anti-A Anti-Rh	Anti-A Anti-Dextran	Anti-Rh	Anti-Rh (few)
Susceptibility to papain cleavage into Fab and Fc	Moderate	Poor	Strong	Moderate

However, under certain conditions some antigens, especially those with a large configuration such as macromolecules or whole cells, can directly stimulate B-cells into antibody production without the aid of T-cell helpers. When this occurs only antibodies of the IgM class are produced with no subsequent switchover to IgG.

Unlike IgG, IgM immunoglobulin does not cross the placenta, partly because of its large size but primarily because its heavy chains do not have a structural characteristic known as the placenta permeability factor. This immunoglobulin is sensitive to reduction by 2-mercaptoethanol, which results in the breaking of disulfide bonds that leads to a depolymerization of the immunoglobulin. Therefore, the agglutinating power of antibodies belonging to the IgM class is destroyed by treatment with this agent. IgG antibodies are not affected by this treatment.

IgA immunoglobulins are of the same relative size as IgG, but very often they autopolymerize into large aggregates having sedimentation coefficients ranging from 7S to 9S for monomers and dimers to 11S for trimers and as high as 19S for very large polymers. Immunoglobulins of this type are present not only in serum, but also in such secreted fluids as nasal secretions, saliva, urine, and meconium, in which case they are known as *secretory IgA*. The chemical composition of secretory IgA is slightly different from serum IgA in that it contains an additional structure known as a *secretory piece* (SP), which confers some unique physicochemical properties on the molecule.

Although circulating antibodies to most of the common blood group antigens are most often thought of as being IgM and IgG, antibodies with corresponding specificities may also be found in secretions. These antibodies belong to the secretory IgA class and as such may play an important role in natural defense mechanisms.

As a rule, antibodies belonging to the IgA class do not cross the placenta in spite of their size, presumably because of the lack of a placenta permeability factor on the Fc fragment. As with other immunoglobulins, the antigenic specificity of IgA itself is conferred by unique structures present in the constant region of the H (α) chains. Treatment with reducing agents such as 2-mercaptoethanol partially inactivates the agglutinating ability of IgA antibodies but does not destroy it completely.

Any discussion of the immunochemistry of antibodies is incomplete without a consideration of antibody heterogeneity and its implications in the use of antisera. Although not emphasized previously, on reaching maturity each plasma cell is capable of producing only one class of heavy chain and one type of light chain having but a single hypervariable region. Therefore, if the antigen, when administered, stimulated only a single cell, a very homogenous population of antibody molecules would be produced. This, however, is not the case. In fact, when an immune response is invoked, a large number of different immunologically competent cells are recruited, each one capable of responding with the production of its own uniquely constructed humoral factor.

Depending on the route of immunization, the dose and characteristics of the antigen, and the immunologic responsiveness of the host, theoretically at least, immunoglobulins of any or perhaps all five major classes, IgM, IgG, IgA, IgD, and IgE, could be produced. The relative amounts of each of these would vary but one class would most likely predominate. In general, IgM is produced as the result of a primary immune response, whereas IgG is the product of a secondary immune response. However, when the challenge presents itself, it is possible that four different classes of γ chains will result, each of which confers particular serologic properties on the final molecule, such as antigen binding, complement activation, and so on. In addition, each of the different antibodies can have either κ light chains or λ light chains contributing to subtly different hypervariable regions in the completed molecules. Finally, consideration must be given to the fact that any antigen found in nature is composed of a number of distinct antigenic determinants. Therefore, a number of cells, each capable of responding to the individual determinants of an antigen, are stimulated into making their products.

During the normal course of events in blood bank work, one normally deals with antisera containing a collection of antibodies rather than with individual antibodies. Therefore, any time that an antiserum directed against a blood group antigen is studied, one must remember that it contains many species of molecules, with subtle differences in specificity and reactivity. The ultimate serologic behavior of such an antiserum as observed in in vitro tests is governed by the most prevalent species of antibody molecules.

CLASSICAL SEROLOGIC PROCEDURES

The most important serologic tool for use in studying blood group antigens and antibodies is the agglutination test. Agglutination is a serologic reaction that is biochemically similar to precipitation except that the antigenic determinants are part of, or attached to, a cell or large insoluble particle rather than being individual molecules in solution. The aggregate that is observed is composed of a latticework in which cells are chemically bound together by means of intercellular bridges of antibody molecules. Because the antigenic carrier is a relatively large particle, very few are needed to form a visible cluster. If one imagines that only a single antibody molecule is needed to unite a pair of cells, it is easy to see that this is one of the most sensitive of all serologic techniques.

As early as 1896, Gruber and Durham observed the clumping of bacteria with specific antisera. Their tests were routinely performed in a menstruum of saline. In other words, the bacterial cells were suspended in physiologic salt solutions, and dilutions of the antiserum were likewise prepared in this medium. Landsteiner's[1] experiments on the agglutination of human red blood cells by isoantibodies were also carried out using saline diluent. In the ensuing thirty years the MN and P blood group systems were discovered by means of saline agglutination reactions and, finally, the original observations of Levine and his coworkers[9] regarding the outcome of similar saline tests eventually led to the discovery of the Rh system. In view of this historic background it is not surprising that the investigators in the field of immunohematology were somewhat astonished to discover that not all agglutinating antibodies could be demonstrated by using physiologic salt solutions as cell-suspending media and antiserum diluents.

The discovery of so-called *incomplete antibodies* in the Rh blood group system ushered in a completely new era in this field. Antibodies of this type have the capacity of combining with their specific antigens either in vivo or in vitro but are not capable of producing visible agglutinations under standard test conditions, i.e., saline diluents. Extensive studies carried out by many investigators have shown that incomplete antibodies can cause the formation of agglutinates if special techniques are used.

Four major techniques have been useful in the detection of incomplete antibodies: the blocking test, the use of colloidal diluents, the pretreatment of the red cells with proteolytic enzymes, and the antiglobulin reaction (Coombs test). The blocking test is included merely for historical interest, as it has since been superceded by more modern methods. However, the underlying principle is still valid and forms the basis for such assays as competitive antibody binding. In this test, erythrocytes carrying the appropriate antigen are first exposed to an antiserum containing an incomplete antibody. After a suitable incubation period, such cells are exposed to another antiserum containing complete antibodies of the same specificity. If the incomplete antibodies in the first serum combine with the antigenic receptor sites on the red cell surface, none remain exposed for combination with the complete antibody in the second antiserum and agglutination cannot take place.

The use of high protein or colloidal substances as red cell suspending agents and antiserum diluents is the simplest method for demonstrating incomplete antibodies. In tests of this type a suitable colloid, such as normal human serum, bovine albumin, high molecular weight dextran, ficol, gelatine, gum acacia, or polyvinylpyrrolidone, is substituted for saline as a diluent. When this is done visible clumps are readily produced by many antibodies of the incomplete variety.

Morton and Pickles[10] pointed out that red cells carrying the appropriate antigens could be agglutinated by an incomplete antibody even when suspended in saline if they had been previously exposed to the action of bacterial filtrates rich in proteolytic enzymes. Since that time the use of purified enzyme preparations, such as bromelin, ficin, trypsin, or papain, has been accepted as a useful serologic method although it is not universally applicable. The technique is complicated by an additional step being involved, and the treatment may damage the antigenic receptor sites of some blood group systems such as MN and Duffy. Nevertheless, some incomplete agglutinins can be demonstrated effectively only by this method.

The exact mode of action of these two methods depends on the fact that they alter the physicochemical conditions that are operative during the second stage of agglutination.

A particularly useful test for the detection of incomplete antibodies is the antiglobulin test developed by Coombs[11] and his coworkers. This test is based on an observation that it is possible to produce an antibody in rabbits that is reactive with human gamma globulin. Such a rabbit antibody will react with any human incomplete antibody attached to a cell surface. Therefore, intercellular bridges made up of rabbit antibodies to gamma globulin can link together red cells coated with human incomplete isoantibodies into large visible aggregates. The principle of the antiglobulin or Coombs test is depicted in Figure 7.

Renton[12] showed that very often certain blood group antibodies that gave no

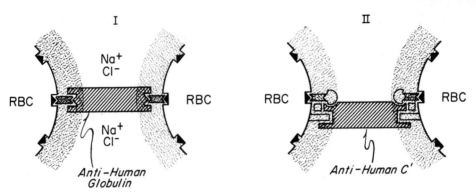

Fig. 7. A diagrammatic representation of the mechanism of agglutinin formation in the two types of antiglobulin reactions. In I, bridges are formed between antibody molecules bound to the surface antigen. In II, bridges are formed between complement components bound as a result of previous antigen-antibody interaction.

reaction with ordinary antiglobulin sera would react if the Coombs reagent (antiwhole human serum) was first neutralized with purified human gamma globulin. They reasoned that the reactive antibody of such neutralized sera was directed against some component of the antigen-antibody system that was basically something other than gamma globulin. Therefore, the term *anti-non-gamma* was originated. It has since been demonstrated that the component involved is complement.

In some systems a much better Coombs reaction can be obtained by making bridges between adjacent complement molecules than between adjacent antibody molecules (Fig. 7). The reasons for this are numerous. Recent evidence suggests that complement is bound directly to the cell membrane. Therefore, it may be that many more, much larger, or much more accessible antigenic sites are offered to the anti-non-gamma Coombs reagent. Furthermore, complement may afford the additional advantage of a stable complex, which cannot be stripped from the cell surface by vigorous washing. The discovery of the various immunoglobulin classes led to the development of immunoglobulin-specific Coombs reagents. Thus, by means of highly selective anti-IgM, anti-IgG, or anti-IgA antisera, the skilled worker can ascertain directly the immunoglobulin class to which a sensitizing antibody belongs. In addition, by the use of certain anticomplement sera of animal origin, it is possible to detect the presence of at least some of the complement components in an antigen-antibody complex that show no evidence of lysis.

The most widely used general purpose antiglobulin serum is the *Broad Spectrum* reagent. This material is usually a specific blend of serum containing antibodies to human γ chains and antibodies to some of the complement components, notably β_{IC}, β_{IE}, and α_{2D}. The ideal blend has not yet been produced as there is some controversy over what its composition should be. Some workers argue that antibodies to other immunoglobulin heavy chains should be included. Others offer various suggestions concerning the relative amounts of antibody needed for each of the complement components to give maximum sensitivity with a minimum of false positives. (Red cells stored as clotted blood in the refrigerator can nonspecifically take up complement.) The experimentalists feel that the broad spectrum concept is unscientific and individual antiglobulin sera should be used, while the more practically oriented claim that exceedingly potent anti-IgG sera will detect all clinically important antibodies that require the antiglobulin technique for their detection.

In the clinical laboratory the antiglobulin test is referred to as the *indirect Coombs test* when it is used to detect the presence of antibody in a patient's serum or if it must be used with a particular typing antiserum for the detection of a certain blood group antigen on red cells. If the antiglobulin test is used to detect the suspected presence of antibody already on the patient's cells, it is referred to as the *direct Coombs test*. Students frequently tend to be confused by this terminology. The essential difference is that the indirect test is a test for antibodies in the serum. Therefore, the cells must be coated, or sensitized, with the primary antibody in the laboratory. The direct test, on the other hand, is a test for antibodies on cells. Therefore, the cells have already been coated in vivo and they need only to be washed to remove unbound protein and treated with the antiglobulin reagent.

PHYSICOCHEMICAL ASPECTS OF AGGLUTINATION

Agglutination is a two-stage phenomenon. In the first step, antibodies combine with the specific antigenic receptor sites on the surface of the carrier particle or cell. During the second stage, the antibody-coated cells, or sensitized cells as they are sometimes called, come together and the antibody molecules combine with additional antigenic receptor sites on other cells, linking them into large aggregates resembling a latticework. It must be emphasized that not only the first stage but also the second stage of this reaction is specific. When a serum containing both anti-A and anti-B antibodies is mixed with a suspension of two populations of cells, one possessing the A antigen and the other possessing the B antigen, two separate types of clumps are formed. One type of clump contains only cells of group A and the other only those of group B (Fig. 8).

The uptake of antibodies in the first stage is a reversible chemical union of the antibody with the antigen on the cell surface that follows the laws of mass action. As such, it reaches equilibrium at some point, depending on the relative concentrations of the reactants and the equilibrium and binding constants of the particular antibody involved. This initial antibody uptake is also affected by the physicochemical conditions of the surrounding medium, the most important of which are temperature, pH, and ionic strength. Ionic strength in particular has a definite effect on the equilibrium constant of some antigen-antibody unions. For instance, a lowering of the ionic strength from 0.15 to 0.07 can cause a considerable increase in the uptake of some incomplete antibodies with a concomitant decrease in the required incubation time.[13]

The rapid antibody uptake achieved with low ionic strength, however, is not observed with all antigen-antibody systems. This may be due either to peculiarities

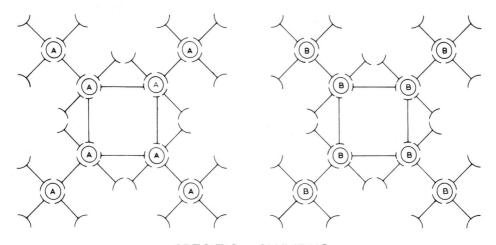

SPECIFIC   CLUMPING

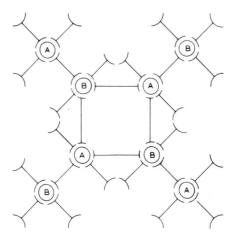

NONSPECIFIC   CLUMPING

Fig. 8. A diagram of the lattice found in aggregates of red cells held together by antibodies showing the types of agglutinates that would be expected with a specific and a nonspecific second-stage reaction. The hybrid clumps are never found.

of the antigenic determinants, such as their individual chemical structure or location on the cell surface, or to peculiarities of the combining site on the antibody, such as the particular sequence, arrangement, or alteration of the amino acids that form the complementary structure, and the immunoglobulin class of the antibody itself.

Temperature can have a profound effect on the final outcome of antigen-antibody reaction. Most antibodies have a particular thermal amplitude or incubation temperature range within which maximum reactions take place. Although the vast majority of human immune alloantibodies react best at body temperature (37C), some require much lower temperatures. The most outstanding of these are the IgM cold agglutinins, which react best at 4C. Antibodies of this type produce aggregates when incubated with red cells at refrigerator temperatures; however, elevating the temperature to 37C results in their complete dispersal.

A difference in thermal amplitude has been used to distinguish *immune antibodies,* those whose production is the result of a definable event, from *naturally occurring antibodies,* those whose production is the result of an undefined universal exposure to ubiquitous antigens. Naturally occurring antibodies usually react better at lower temperatures (20C) than at body temperature. Exactly the reverse is true of those agglutinins produced as a result of specific immunization.

The second stage of agglutination consists of the specific formation of aggregates. This is accomplished by means of intercellular antibody bridges. Under normal conditions, red cells in suspension have a net negative surface charge. Because like charges repel one another, red cells in suspension normally stay apart a certain distance, governed by their effective net surface charge density. When cells are suspended in electrolytes the ions in solution orient themselves about the surface of the cell. The orientation of these ions becomes more diffuse as the distance from the cell surface increases. As the cells float through the medium, some of these ions travel with them. Thus, the cells are said to be surrounded by a diffuse double layer or *ionic cloud.* The outer edge of this layer is called the *surface of shear.* These layers are shown diagrammatically in Figure 9. There is a difference in electrostatic potential between the net charge at the cell membrane and the charge at the surface of shear; therefore, an electrostatic potential exists between these two points—the zeta potential. The zeta potential is dependent on the actual net surface charge density at the surface of the cell membrane and the dielectric constant and ionic strength of the surrounding medium.

The formation of aggregates during the second stage of agglutination requires that a cell with an antibody attached to its surface approach another cell close enough to permit the antibody molecule to bridge the gap and combine with the antigenic site on the second cell. When the electrostatic forces involved are sufficiently strong, cells can never come close enough to each other to allow the chemical binding and resultant lattice formation to take place (Fig. 10).

In many agglutination systems, the problems of distance between adjacent cells can be partially overcome by subjecting the cells to high gravitational forces in a centrifuge, thereby counteracting repulsive effects and forcing the cells together. However, some antibody molecules, notably the incomplete variety of IgG, can

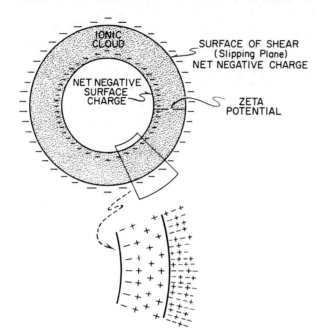

Fig. 9. Schematic representation of the electrical charges surrounding a particle in suspension. (Adapted from Pollack et al. *Transfusion* 5:158, 1965.)

never bridge the gap unless extremely high gravitational forces are employed. The magnitude of the gravitational forces required is often impractical for routine work.

The exact distance required for optimum agglutination will vary according to the antigen-antibody system involved. The distance is dependent not only on the size of the antibody molecule produced but also on the particular location of the antigenic receptor site in relation to the effective surface.

Pollack[14] has suggested that it is possible to alter electrostatically imposed intercellular distances and, therefore, effect agglutination with incomplete IgG antibodies merely by altering the zeta potential. Two principal techniques are used to alter the zeta potential. One of these is to change the dielectric constant of the medium by using various colloidal solutions, such as bovine albumin, as cell-suspending agents and antibody diluents. The efficiency of a particular diluent in bringing about visible agglutination with incomplete antibodies depends on its own particular ability to alter the dielectric constant. This ability may not always be proportional to the concentration of the material but rather to the chemical properties and composition of the colloid.

Care must be exercised in using any of these special diluents, for it is possible to sufficiently change the physical environment to such an extent that nonspecific aggregation, even without antibodies, will take place. Exactly this principle is employed in some of the automated agglutination techniques.[15] Cells are first exposed to antibodies at low ionic strengths, permitting maximum antibody uptake, and then are caused to hyperaggregate with the aid of high molecular weight polymers.

Another and perhaps more direct method of altering the zeta potential is by a mild treatment of the erythrocytes with proteolytic enzymes such as trypsin, ficin,

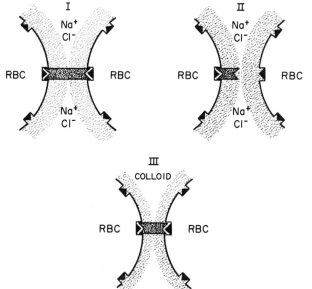

Fig. 10. A schematic diagram showing Pollack's theory applied to agglutination with complete antibodies (**I**) and incomplete antibodies (**II** and **III**). The shaded areas represent the magnitude or the electrostatic forces in effect at the red cell surface. Complete antibodies of the IgM class have a greater effective length and can bridge the distance between two cells in spite of maximum electrostatic effects. Incomplete IgG can bridge only when these effects are minimized.

bromelin, or papain. This treatment physically reduces the cells' net surface charge density by removing surface sialic acid residues, thereby effectively lowering the zeta potential. Unfortunately, as mentioned previously, the antigenic determinants of certain blood group systems are extremely susceptible to this treatment and can be destroyed or stripped off the cell with such enzymes. Therefore, enzymatic pretreatment cannot be employed as a routine technique and should be used only with the appropriate controls.

ELUTION

The knowledge of the effects of various physical conditions on antibody uptake can be a very valuable tool for the serologist. For example, since the combination of an antibody with its antigen is a reversible chemical reaction, an alteration of the physical conditions associated with the reaction can result in a release of the antibody. This is a phenomenon referred to as elution. The technique of elution is often used for preparing serologically pure antibodies according to the flow chart shown in Figure 11. Suppose that one has a serum containing antibodies that react well at 37C but are directed against several antigenic determinants. The serum can be mixed with a suspension of cells that have only that antigenic determinant for which pure antibodies are desired. After incubation, the suspension is washed free of uncombined antibodies and subjected to an increased temperature, a decreased pH, or a change in ionic strength. Under these adverse conditions the antigen-antibody complex will break, and antibodies of the single specificity will be released

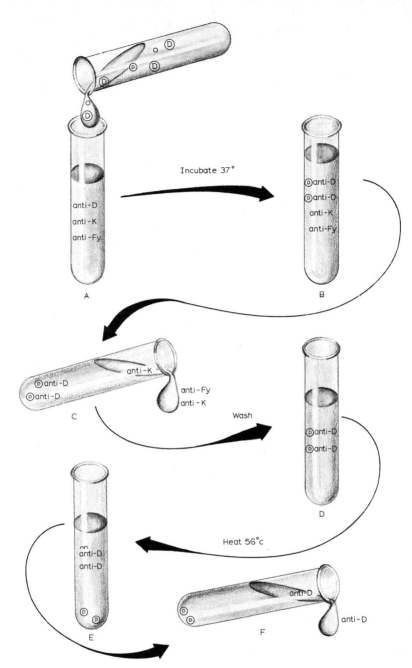

Fig. 11. An example of antibody purification by elution. **A.** Red cells containing only the antigens that correspond to the specificity that is to be purified are added to the serum containing the antibody mixture. In this case the specificity is D. **B.** During incubation the anti-D antibodies bind to the D-positive red cells, while the others remain free. **C.** After centrifuging the red cells, the unwanted antibodies can be removed by decanting and further washing. **D.** This leaves only the anti-D antibodies bound to the red cells. **E.** Heating the suspension breaks the antigen-antibody complex, releasing pure anti-D into the supernatant or eluate. **F.** The eluate containing antibodies can be decanted after centrifugation.

into the surrounding medium. Such a preparation is known as an *eluate* and is frequently very useful in the study of certain immunologic phenomena.

COMPLEMENT IN ANTIGEN-ANTIBODY REACTIONS

In serologic tests involving erythrocytes, it is imperative to be aware of the complement system and its mode of action. First, one should realize that hemolysis of the test cells is as much an endpoint of an antigen-antibody reaction as is agglutination. Second, as already discussed, broad spectrum antihuman globulin reagents contain anticomplement component antibodies (usually anti-C3 and anti-C4). These antibodies will react with their specific cell-bound complement components whether the blood group specific antibodies that initially bond to red cell membrane antigens are present or not. Thus even though the antibody that caused the complement activation may have been eluted from the cells either deliberately or accidentally, or if the components were membrane-bound through some antibody independent mechanism, positive reactions using such antiglobulin reagents can still occur.

Some of the complement components are heat-labile, being destroyed by a temperature of 56C for thirty minutes. In addition, however, they have a rapid normal decay rate even at 4C, so that the minimum level of complement activity needed to detect complement-binding antibodies is reached in a short period of time. Thus, complement activity disappears as a result of aging upon storage unless extremely low temperatures are used to retard the process.

Complement (C) is a complex system of serum proteins that can participate in a variety of serologic reactions, not all of which result in the lysis of cells.

In addition to cell lysis, key elements of the system are important in various kinds of enhanced immunologically directed responses such as vascular permeability, immune adherence, conglutination, complement-mediated phagocytosis, chemotaxis, cytotoxicity, and cytolysis, as well as the release of histamine and lysosomal enzymes responsible for tissue damage. Many of the components of this system have been isolated and are well-described proteins: the majority are beta globulins that circulate in the plasma in an inactive native form. This circulating resting state is referred to as the fluid phase.

At the present time eleven major components of the classical complement system have been identified and numbered C1 through C9. Their properties are listed in Table 4. Most complement components are cleaved into subcomponents when the native or fluid phase component is activated. For example, C1, the first component, is a macromolecule that is composed of three subunits, C1q, C1r, and C1s.* Some subcomponents are enzymes that participate directly in the lytic sequence, while others participate in the additional biologic functions of the complement system.

---

* Activated forms are distinguished from their inactive counterparts by a bar over the component number (eg C$\overline{1}$) and the subunits are identified by the addition of lower case letters (eg C$\overline{1}$q).

TABLE 4. COMPONENTS AND SUBUNITS OF THE COMPLEMENT SYSTEM

Component	Electro-phoretic Mobility	Serum Concen-tration (g/ml)	Comments
C1	γ_2		Subunits held together by Ca++
C1q (1 mole)	γ_2	180	Reacts with Fc fragment of bound antibody
C1r (2 mole)	β_1	100	
C1s (4 mole)	α_2	80	Enzymatic activity for C4 and C2
C4	β_1	450	Cleaved by C1s
C4a			Remains in plasma
C4b			Cell-bound
C2	β_1	25	Attaches to cell-bound C4b in presence of Mg^{++} cleaved by C1s
C2a			Remains with C4b to form C4b2A (C3 convertase)
C2b			Released to plasma
C3	β_2	1500	Cleaved by C3 convertase (C4b2a)
C3a			Anaphylatotoxin; remains in plasma
C3b	β_1E		Cell-bound, adjacent to C4b2a to form C4b2a3b
C3c	β_1A		Acted on by C3 inactivator (C3INA) to form C3c and C3d
C3d	α_2D		Cell-bound, biologically inactive
C5	β_1	75	Cleaved by C4b2a3b, last enzymatic step
C5a			Anaphylatotoxin; remains in plasma
C5b			Cell-bound to C4b2a3b5b complex
C6	β_2	60	Binds to C4b2a3b5b
C7	β_2	60	Binds to C5b6 (C5b67) complex, can move to new membrane site
C8	γ_1	80	Binds to C5b67 complex
C9	α	150	Binds to C8 (up to 6 molecules)

The activation of various complement components, which may eventually lead to hemolysis by producing minute holes in the erythrocyte membrane, is a step-like chain of events. For the most part, the complement system is an interdependent enzymatic system, composed of activators and inactivators, in which each succeeding component is activated by the preceding one. Thus, the activation sequence is a cascade similar to the one operative in the coagulation mechanism. This analogy goes beyond merely a striking similarity in cascade effect. There is evidence that the complement and the coagulation system can interact. It is thought that this interaction of the two systems accounts for the disruption of normal hemostatis that may occasionally accompany immunologically caused hemolytic transfusion reactions.

In immunohematology, the lytic action of complement brought about through the classical pathway is the most important. The actual lysis of cells is the direct result of complement action rather than antibodies. An antibody coupled to antigen merely serves to activate the complement system. The activation, fixation, or binding of complement may be accomplished most effectively by IgM, IgG1, IgG2, or IgG3 antibodies as a result of complement activator groups located on the Fc fragments of their heavy chains. The immunoglobulins IgA, IgD, and IgE are not known to bind complement. The effectiveness of IgM in producing complement-mediated hemolysis is twice that of IgG. Thus, for complement binding to take place only one antibody molecule is needed if it is IgM; while two antibody molecules are required if it is IgG. The reason for this is that two adjacent Fc fragments are necessary to bind $C\overline{1q}$. Therefore, monomeric antibody molecules such as IgG with but one Fc fragment per molecule must attach to two adjacent receptor sites. A single IgM antibody being a pentamer, on the other hand, has ten combining sites and five Fc fragments associated with each molecule; therefore, a reaction of this antibody with but a single antigenic receptor site is adequate to furnish the required pair of closely associated Fc fragments needed to activate complement. It is possible that this is one of the reasons why many blood group antibodies fail to activate complement. For example, if the distribution of a certain antigenic receptor site on the cell surface is sparse and the antibody regularly produced against it is of the IgG type, we would expect homolysis to be an unusual event. The physical proximity of the activator Fc fragments is one of the most significant requirements, and there is evidence suggesting that the two IgG molecules necessary for activating complement need not even be directed against the same antigen. This is an important consideration, especially when studying the lytic properties of sera containing antibodies with a variety of specificities.

Complement can be activated whenever appropriate antibody binding with antigenic receptor sites takes place. As a direct result of such binding a complex series of events, shown schematically in Figure 12, takes place. First, some change is effected in the Fc region of the antibody molecule so that it is capable of activating C1 proesterase and subsequently combining with the resultant $C\overline{1q}$ esterase. The reaction of the antibody with its antigen merely alters the Fc fragment so that it can activate and accept a $C\overline{1q}$ molecule; the actual attachment, however, is due to random chance, rather than some type of chemotactic effect. Further, C1 is not firmly bound to the Fc fragment and, therefore, it can dissociate from one antibody molecule and attach to another. With activation of $C\overline{1q}$, the other C1 subunits, $C\overline{1r}$ and $C\overline{1s}$, become activated and form a stable complex held together with the aid of Ca^{++}.

C1 (specifically $C\overline{1s}$) activates C4, which is split into subunits $C\overline{4a}$ and $C\overline{4b}$. $C\overline{4a}$ remains in the plasma while $C\overline{4b}$ attaches directly to the cell surface. C2 subsequently attached to $C\overline{4b}$ in the presence of Mg^{++}, is acted on by $C\overline{1s}$, and cleaved into subunits $C\overline{2a}$ and $C\overline{2b}$. $C\overline{2a}$ remains attached to the cell-bound $C\overline{4b}$ molecule, thereby completing the formation of the $C\overline{4b2a}$ complex, which is also called C3 convertase. This complex is an enzyme that activates native C3, with resultant formation of $C\overline{3a}$ and $C\overline{3b}$. $C\overline{3b}$ becomes cell-bound at another membrane site and associates with $C\overline{4b2a}$, forming the $C\overline{4b2a3b}$ complex known as C5 convertase. This substance in turn activates native C5, resulting in the formation of $C\overline{5a}$ and $C\overline{5b}$. The activation of C5 appears to be the last enzymatic step. $C\overline{5b}$ binds to the $C\overline{4b2a3b}$ complex, to which C6 and C7 then attach. The $C\overline{5b67}$ com-

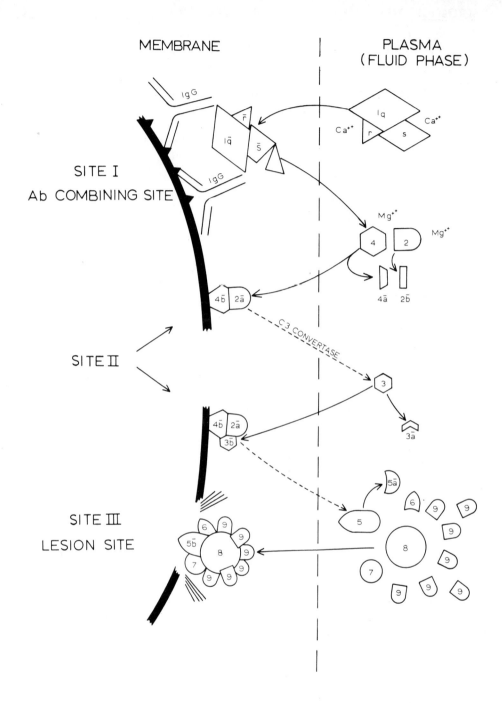

Fig. 12. The cascading steps involved in the activation and binding of the various components of complement. (Adapted from Müller-Eberhard et al. *Arch Pathol* 82:205, 1966.)

plex is actually a subcomplex that can dissociate from the major complex and reattach to a different site on the membrane. C8 becomes attached to the $\overline{C5b,6,7}$ complex, and finally C9 binds to C8.

Cell membrane damage begins to occur immediately upon the attachment of $\overline{C5b67}$. Lysis itself begins slowly with the addition of C8, but progresses rapidly when C9 enters the reaction. By a still unexplained mechanism, a holelike alteration of about 10 nm is produced in the cell membrane, allowing the cytoplasmic contents to spill.

This chain of events is a simplified version of the process as it is currently understood.[16] Each enzyme that is formed has the potential of activating many molecules of the next component. Only a portion of these takes part in the reaction, while many become inactive and no longer participate. A single antigen-antibody reaction can result in exponential activation of complement components, thus amplifying the effect of the original antigen-antibody reaction.

SEROLOGIC TESTS OF THE FUTURE

Miniaturization

The miniaturization of serologic tests originated with the workers in the field of human lymphocyte typing, a topic to be touched on in a subsequent chapter. Basically, these workers were faced with the double problem of a chronic shortage of suitable antibodies and the small number of lymphocytes in the peripheral blood. As a result, they scaled down serologic tests so that routinely as little as 1 μl of antiserum could be used with as few as 2,000 cells. Since the ordinary test tubes used in serologic work could not be employed with such minuscule volumes of materials, special plates containing reaction wells adaptable to microscopic evaluation were developed. In addition, routine pipettes were replaced with mechanically operated repeating syringelike dispensers.

Miniaturization has several advantages beyond those of reagent conservation. The newer technology permits the tests to be set up rapidly and accurately. Since there is no need to bother with cumbersome tubes and racks, it is simple to arrange the work in a format that permits data collection and analysis by computer. Finally, the possibility of complete automation of reading, interpretation, and reporting becomes very real.

Some attempts at reducing the scale of blood bank serology have been made already. For example, the capillary agglutination method of Chown, which antedates the lymphocyte typing era by at least a decade or more, has been used sporadically over the years by a few workers. In this method a red cell suspension is mixed with antiserum contained in a capillary tube and the tube is incubated in an inclined position. Cells that react with the antibodies form aggregates that settle more rapidly than cells that do not react. By measuring the degree of settling in a given time period it is possible to distinguish positives from negatives. This technique was originally introduced to conserve precious Rh reagents but has since proved to be a highly sensitive method for detecting certain incomplete agglutinins. At present it is enjoying a renewal as a possible alternative to more cumbersome methods.[17]

Agglutination in microtiter plates was introduced a number of years ago. Microtiter plates are plastic trays with ninety-six molded wells, each capable of holding about 20 μl. The geometry of the wells is such that very small volumes of antisera and red cells can be employed successfully. The final reactions can be observed, macroscopically, microscopically, or nephelometrically and the plate wells can be easily photographed for future reference. All procedures normally performed in test tubes can be carried out with equal facility in microtiter plates. As yet this method has not gained widespread popularity.[18]

TESTS BASED ON ANTIBODY BINDING

As discussed previously, agglutination is a two-stage phenomenon. As a result it is plagued with the problems that are associated with the lattice-forming step. Therefore, unless the test environment is such that lattice formation can take place, it is impossible to tell whether or not a reaction has occurred regardless of the degree of the primary antigen-antibody reaction.

This disadvantage can be overcome by using an assay system that directly measures the presence of an antibody bound to an antigen. Such a system offers an additional advantage in that it is possible to measure the amount of antibodies with varying degrees of precision and therefore, possibly, the amount of antigen present on the cell.

Two systems are presently in the developmental stages and, as with miniaturization, they offer the advantages of automation and direct computer interfacing for data processing. The first of these is a direct radioimmunoassay RIA, introduced by Masouredis a number of years ago. It involves the use of an antiglobulin serum that is radiolabeled with ^{125}I. Briefly, in the test system cells are incubated with the antiserum in question and then washed free of unbound antibodies. The radioactive antiglobulin serum is then added, incubated, and excess material washed off. The amount of radioactivity present on the surface is determined by measurement in a gamma counter. This value can be extrapolated to represent the number of antibody molecules bound. A number of variations on this system have been devised, the best being one in which a highly purified specific immunoglobulin preparation is labeled with an isotope directly. The single most significant disadvantage of any of these methods is the fact that a radioisotope must be used.

Another method designed to measure antibody binding is the ELISA (enzyme linked immunosorbant assay) method. This technique was introduced in the late 1970s, and in 1980 Perkins applied it to blood grouping problems.[19] As with the indirect RIA, this technique makes use of an antiglobulin reagent. However, in this case the antiglobulin is coupled to an active enzyme such as alkaline phosphatase. After the reaction is completed and appropriate washes performed, the linked enzyme's substrate, in this case p-nitrophenyl phosphate, is added and an assay is performed to assess the color change resulting from the enzymatic cleavage of free phosphate. This may be only a matter of examining the tubes or titration plates for the presence or absence of color. The test can be quantitated by reading the density of the color in a spectrophotometer.

All binding assays, but especially the indirect assays, depend on the availability of highly specific antibodies to the antigen in question. Since all indicators of binding are nonspecific with respect to the antigen on the red cell, they will combine with all antibody molecules that are attached to any antigen on the cell surface. To some extent this requirement excludes the use of the kinds of alloantisera that are routinely employed in blood banks, since as was noted earlier an alloantibody response results in the production of a large variety of antibody molecules, each bearing a highly specific but different specificity. In the experimental lab this problem is overcome by the use of reagents that have been highly purified by various immunochemical methods based on sophisticated techniques of elution. The cost of such reagents up until now has been prohibitive for routine use.

Another new technology has been introduced recently that will make exceedingly pure reagents in plentiful supply and, it is hoped, at a reasonable cost. This is the method of in vitro monoclonal antibody production.[20, 21] In this technique, specific antibody-producing cells are genetically fused with myeloma cells growing in tissue culture. The antibody-producing cells have the genetic information required for the production of a certain hypervariable region of an antibody molecule. The myeloma cells, on the other hand, are malignant cells that reproduce readily and are capable of making huge quantities of immunoglobulins. The result of such a fusion is a cell possessing the high immunoglobulin production potential of a malignant cell that has been genetically instructed to make an immunoglobulin bearing a particular antibody specificity.

After such a fusion, individual cells making the desired antibody are selected by screening and are cloned. All of the cells in such a clone make very large amounts of only one kind of antibody that reacts with a single antigenic determinant. Although this era is only beginning, a time can be foreseen when such reagents, used in fully automated binding assays and interfaced with computers, will be routinely employed in most modern blood bank laboratories (Fig. 13).

BLOOD-GROUPING REAGENTS

The reagents used in blood bank laboratories, both antisera and test cells, are commercially available from a number of reputable diagnostic reagent manufacturers. These reagents are manufactured under federal licensure according to rigid specifications established and enforced by the Bureau of Biologics. The fact that the reagents are manufactured under license ensures the user that they can be expected to perform according to a defined set of minimum standards.[22]

Although each reagent must be shown to meet minimum requirements for activity, some variation may be observed among the products of various manufacturers. Therefore, even though all of them meet the basic criteria some may exceed those criteria. For this reason most laboratories expend considerable effort to com-

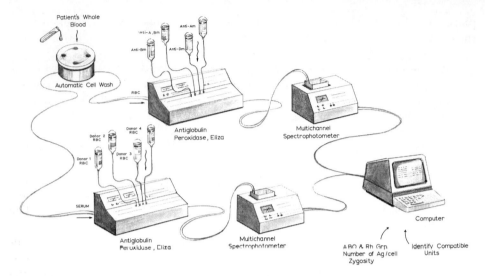

Fig. 13. The automated blood bank of the future will depend on monoclonal antibodies and sensitive spectrophotometric binding assays. In this rendition, a small blood sample can be tested automatically for its red cell and serum properties as well as cross-matched with suitable donors. The final results are analyzed and sorted by an on-line computer.

pare various reagents and select those that give optimal results in their own hands. Although they may not be as necessary today as they were in the past, some comparative studies are still worthwhile, especially when reagents are uncommon or when laboratory conditions present unusual problems.

Most blood-grouping sera are manufactured from the plasma of people who have been alloimmunized as a result of transfusion or pregnancy. In some cases volunteers are immunized deliberately to increase their levels of alloantibodies to make their plasma a more useful source of raw material.

The finished product is usually different from the original serum containing antibodies in its composition and even its appearance. (Anti-A reagent is normally colored blue-green and anti-B colored yellow so that they may be easily distinguished.) Apart from this many sera undergo extensive purification and other steps to make them usable as reagents. In some cases the antibodies are purified and resuspended in artificial diluents, which stabilize them and enhance their activity in various serologic tests. Sometimes antibody activities of various specificities from different sources are scientifically blended to produce a finished reagent that will perform in accordance with design specifications. The production of each reagent is carefully monitored during the manufacturing process by testing it with appropriate red cells according to specific serologic techniques. Finally, the finished product is always accompanied by an instruction brochure spelling out in considerable detail the method to be employed in its use. Any deviation from the prescribed method can result in false reactivity of the reagent, which will lead to erroneous and sometimes dangerous results. All users of commercially prepared blood-grouping reagents are cautioned to read direction circulars very carefully and to abide by all of the manufacturer's suggested methods.

Commercial antisera can be divided into several categories, depending on the techniques to be employed for their use. The most commonly available are called *Slide* or *Rapid Tube.* As the names imply, these reagents are intended for slide tests or tube tests that are not normally incubated. In general, such reagents are manufactured from IgG immunoglobulin, which is an incomplete antibody. With few exceptions they are used with red cells, as they are found in unseparated whole blood. The native serum of whole blood behaves as the enhancing agent and allows visible agglutination to occur. Since red cells need not be separated from the serum and since the antibodies themselves have a very strong affinity (high binding) and avidity (bind quickly), the test can be performed rapidly.

The use of reagents of this type is common in most clinical laboratories. Certain precautions, however, must be taken to ensure the quality of the result. Since the antibodies used are IgG, which require high protein fortifiers found in the reagents themselves as well as in the serum of the test cells, false positive reactions can be obtained if the red cells of the individual being tested are already coated with incomplete antibodies. This might be the case, for example, in patients who have an immune autoantibody type of acquired hemolytic anemia. The agglutination that occurs when such blood is mixed with a Slide or Rapid Tube reagent can be caused by either the specific blood group reactivity or the nonspecific autoagglutination induced by the antiserum diluent. Therefore, whenever such reagents are used they must be accompanied by a control consisting of the diluent the manufacturer used in making the reagent. In view of this need, many manufacturers supply such diluents as companions to their blood-grouping sera. It must be stressed, however, that due to differences in formulation from one manufacturer to the next, the control and the reagent must be obtained from the same source. Interchanging manufacturers in this step must be avoided.

Another group of reagents are those labeled *Saline Tube Test.* As the name implies these reagents are to be used with washed red cells suspended in saline. Reagents of this type are made from IgM antibodies or certain IgG antibodies that normally produce visible agglutination without the aid of an enhancing agent. Antibodies of this type are less avid and require various periods of incubation at 37 C. Again, the time and temperature are specified by the manufacturer and must be adhered to strictly.

The sera from which these reagents are manufactured frequently contain antibodies of other specificities that are IgG and behave as incomplete antibodies. Although every effort is usually made in the manufacturing process to remove these antibodies, some may still be left behind. Therefore, if such reagents are used in slide or rapid tube methods or by the antiglobulin (Coombs) techniques, these antibodies will have an opportunity to react and give false positive results.

There is yet another group of blood-grouping antisera that must be used by the indirect antiglobulin technique. For the most part it is prudent though not completely necessary to use an antiglobulin serum manufactured by the same firm as that which produced the typing reagent. One of the principle reasons for this suggestion is that any producer of a typing serum employs its own antiglobulin sera in the manufacture and standardization of the final typing product, although most manufacturers test their finished products with antiglobulin sera from a number of sources in anticipation of their use in the field.

Finally, a new generation of blood-grouping reagents has been introduced recently. These are reagents that afford the high speed and avidity of test tube reagents with the superb specificity of saline reagents and at a lower cost. They can be considered as artificial reagents made from IgG antibodies that are chemically treated to partially cleave and open the disulfide bridge. This increases the effective length of the molecule and allows it to undergo lattice formation in electrolyte solution. This group of reagents, because of its unique nature, must be used exactly as specified.

Antiglobulin sera come in a variety of different compositions ranging from broad spectrum to those specific for a single immunoglobulin class or complement component. It is possible to obtain specific anti-IgG, anti-IgM, anti-IgA as well as anti-C3 antiglobulin sera from commercial sources. Each of these has a particular place in the laboratory, governed by the function that needs to be accomplished.

For example, for blood-grouping work in an indirect test with most commercially available typing sera a pure anti-IgG reagent may be most useful. For the most part, commercial typing sera to be used in this method are IgG antibodies, and complement is rarely involved. For antibody identification and cross-matching, on the other hand, most investigators recommend the use of broad spectrum reagents. Such antiglobulin sera contain antibodies to most of the significant immunoglobulin classes as well as to certain complement components. Because in the application of the antiglobulin reaction the class of the antibody in question is unknown, this seems like a logical approach. Although certain highly specific and potent examples of anti-IgG antiglobulin reagents are capable of detecting all varieties of incomplete antibody, they are not generally available for routine use. Consequently, the broad spectrum approach is currently the most practical.

When the direct antiglobulin reaction is to be used for the diagnosis of autoimmune acquired hemolytic anemia, immunoglobulin and complement-specific reagents are useful since they can give the clinician some clue as to the pathogenesis and possible treatment of the disease.

Reagent selection is a major decision in any blood bank laboratory. The type of reagent to be used is dictated by the type of service being offered as well as the patient population. Those reagents used in a primary care facility would not necessarily be the same as those required in a tertiary care teaching institution. In any event the final decision should be based on knowledge and experience.

Review Questions

1. Antibodies of which immunoglobulin classes are most affected by the addition of 2-mercaptoethanol?
2. List three distinctive features of IgG, IgM, and IgA.
3. What portion of an antibody molecule is associated with antigen binding?

4. What portion of an antibody molecule contributes to its biological function?
5. Name the immunoglobulin class to which incomplete antibodies usually belong.
6. Which complement complex requires calcium ions to maintain its integrity?
7. What antibodies can be detected rapidly by enzyme techniques?
8. What is complement?
9. How long will it usually take before the primary response to $D(Rh_o)$ antigen is detectable?
10. List several causes for a false negative antiglobulin test.
11. List reasons for a false positive antiglobulin test.
12. What is the serologic reaction employed in most blood bank tests?
13. Describe the characteristic features of a secondary immune response.
14. How is antihuman serum prepared from rabbit serum?
15. Describe the phenomenon of cross-reactivity.
16. Describe the general chemical and biological properties of an antigen.
17. What is a hapten?

REFERENCES

1. Landsteiner K: Ueber agglutinationserscheinungen normalen menschlichen Blutes. Wien Klin Wochenschr 14:1132, 1901.
2. Feldman JD: Ultrastructure of immunologic process. Adv Immunol 4:175, 1964.
3. Landsteiner K and van der Scheer J: Serological differentiation of steric isomers (antigens containing tartaric acids). J Exp Med 50:407, 1929.
4. Edelman GM: Antibody structure and molecular immunology. Ann NY Acad Sci 190:5, 1971.
5. Poljak RJ: X-ray studies of immunoglobulins. Adv Immunol 21:1, 1975.
6. Natvig JB and Kunkel HC: Human immunoglobulins: Classes, subclasses, genetic variants, and idiotypes. Adv Immunol 16:1, 1973.
7. Svehag SE, Chesebro B, and Bloth B: Electron microscopy of virus-IgM antibody complexes and free IgM immunoglobulins. Gamma Globulins, Proc Third Nobel Symp. New York, Interscience, 1967, p 269.
8. Eisen HN: Antibody structure: the immunoglobulin. In Davis BD, Dulbecco R, Eisen HN, Ginsberg HS, Wood WB (eds): Microbiology. 2nd ed. Hagerstown, Md, Harper, 1973, p 430.
9. Levine P, Katzin EM, and Burnham L: Isoimmunization in pregnancy, its possible bearing on the etiology and erythroblastosis foetalis. JAMA 116:825, 1941.
10. Morton JA and Pickles MM: The use of trypsin in the detection of incomplete anti-Rh antibodies. Nature 159:779, 1947.
11. Coombs RRA, Mourant AE, and Race PR: A new test for the detection of weak and "incomplete" Rh agglutinins. Br J Exp Pathol 26:255, 1945.
12. Renton PH: Separation of Coombs reagents into two fractions. Nature 169:329, 1952.

13. Moore HC and Mollison PL: Use of low-ionic-strength medium in manual tests for antibody detection. Transfusion 16:291, 1976.

14. Pollack W and Reckel RP: A reappraisal of the zeta potential model of hemagglutination in human blood groups. Mohn JF, Plunkett RW, Cummingham RK, and Lambert (eds): 5th Int Convoc Immunol 1976. Basel, Karger, 1977, p 17.

15. Rosenfield RE, Szymanski IO, and Kochwa S: Automated methods for the detection and measurement of hemagglutinins. Proc Xth Cong Int Soc Blood Transfusion, Stockholm, 1964.

16. Mayer M: The complement system. Sci Am 229:54, 1973.

17. Crawford MN, Gottman FE, and Rogers LC: Capillary tube testing and enhancement with 30% albumin. Vox Sang 30:144, 1976.

18. McCloskey RV and Zmijewski CM: A semi-microtechnic for the detection of human blood group isohemagglutinins. Am J Clin Pathol 48:240, 1967.

19. Leikola J and Perkins HA: Red cells antibodies and low ionic strength: A study with enzyme-linked antiglobulin test. Transfusion 20:224, 1980.

20. Kennett RH, McKearn TJ, and Bechtol K: Monoclonal Antibodies, Hybridomas: A New Dimension in Biological Analyses. New York, Plenum Press, 1980.

21. Voak D, Sacks S, Alderson T, Takei F, Lennox E, Jarvis J, Milstein C, and Darnborough J: Monoclonal anti-A from a hybrid-myeloma: Evaluation as a blood grouping reagent. Vox Sang 39:134, 1980.

22. Code of Federal Regulations: Title 21 Food and Drugs, Pts. 600–1299—Rev. 1 April 1980. Washington, DC, U.S. Government Printing Office, 1980.

CHAPTER 5

Blood Group Systems

Objectives

From the information presented in this chapter the student should learn the:
1. Basic laws of Mendelian genetics.
2. Mathematical and statistical manipulations used in the solution of genetic problems.
3. Introductory concepts of statistical methods and their application to blood group serology.
4. Fundamentals of the chi-square test.
5. Basic definition of a blood group system.
6. Features of the clinically significant blood group systems, including the nomenclature for the antigens and the characteristic serologic behavior of the specific antibodies.
7. General population frequencies of the major antigens.
8. Alternate nomenclatures used in the Rh system.
9. Physiologic mechanisms associated with hemolytic disease of the newborn.

GENETICS USED IN BLOOD GROUPS

All blood group alloantigens are inherited characteristics under genetic control. As such they conform to the general laws of heredity originally set forth by Gregor Mendel. This Augustinian monk coupled astute observation with mathematical reasoning to formulate and establish the principles that form the foundation of modern genetics. These principles can be summarized in five key statements:

1. There are particles governing hereditary traits which are passed on from one generation to the next.
2. Each individual contains two such particles for each trait; these, however, segregate at gamete formation, only one of each pair going to a single gamete (The Law of Segregation).
3. An individual containing two unlike particles for a given trait may show only the effect of one of these (The Concept of Dominance). This does not affect their transmission to the next generation.
4. The assortment of a pair of these particles is independent of the other pairs (The Law of Independent Assortment). Thus the presence of the particles in a single gamete results from random distribution of the particles contained in the individual.
5. The results of matings are describable in terms of mathematical probability.

Contemporary knowledge dictates that hereditary information concerning physical characteristics apart from those contributing to sex differences is passed on from generation to generation by bits of nucleic acid (DNA) sequences that form the twenty-two pairs of autosomal chromosomes. These bits of genetic information are known as *Genes,* and every individual carries two genes for each attribute, one transmitted by the maternal ovum or *female gamete* and the other passed on from the paternal spermatozoan or *male gamete.*

Through an exceedingly slow and natural process, the genes for a given characteristic undergo spontaneous evolutionary change. This process, referred to as *mutation,* results in the development of alternate forms for each of the genes. These alternate forms are called *alleles.* The consequence of such natural mutation with resultant allelism is the basis for the variety observed in nature of intraspecies characteristics, such as the pigmentation of the eyes, hair, and skin, stature, and physical form as well as a host of less visible biochemical structures, among which are the blood groups. The existence of a variety of a particular attribute within a species is referred to as *polymorphism.*

If an individual inherits an identical allele for a given form of a certain factor from each parent he or she is said to be *homozygous,* or to have a double dose of the gene. If each parent contributes a different allele the individual is *heterozygous* for the characteristic and has a single dose of each gene.

In certain genetic systems, the products formed as a result of the action of one allele, i.e., its phenotypic expression, may mask the presence of the other allele. The allele that can be discerned, whether it is homozygous or heterozygous, is referred to as dominant, whereas the alternate is recessive. The products of recessive genes can be observed only when the individual is homozygous for the appropriate recessive allele or whenever the dominant allele is absent. The simplest case and the one that usually applies to routine blood group serology is the one in which alleles complying with the genetic definition of recessive are *amorphs*. These are genes that appear to have no detectable products and may be encountered especially in those systems in which the formation of a given blood group specificity is the consequence of a complex biochemical pathway involving sequential enzymatic action. The lack of an appropriate enzyme due to the presence of an amorph results in the failure to transform a particular substrate into a given antigenic specificity. On the other hand, if at least one dominant allele is present, the appropriate enzyme is formed, the substrate is converted, and the antigen is produced.

For the most part, the majority of the genes controlling the serologic specificity of the blood group antigens behave as dominant, since each gene results in the formation of a detectable product. However, individuals who are homozygous for given alleles in some of the systems that have been described exhibit quantitatively more antigen on their cell surface then those who are heterozygous. Therefore, such antigens are said to be dose dependent.

The actual genetic makeup of an individual is referred to as a *genotype*. The collection of observable features, on the other hand, is referred to as a *phenotype*. In blood-grouping work, because of the phenomenon of codominance, the observed phenotype of discernible antigens in most blood group systems is frequently the same as the genotype. This phenomenon makes these characteristics very useful in genetic and forensic applications.

The spot on a chromosome where genetic information regulating a particular phenotypic attribute is situated is called a *locus*. At one time it was felt that only a single gene could occupy a locus. However, present genetic thinking does not allow for a finite structural limit for the gene. The more modern concept holds that a locus may not be a precise structure and it can in effect contain several genes and be more accurately considered a gene complex.

During the formation of gametes by the process of meiotic cell division, when the chromosome number is reduced to one half of the total, the chromosome pairs twist and bend before separating. In the course of this process the chromosomal DNA strands can break and recombine (Fig. 1). Because of the accurate alignment of the chromosomes during this step, the breaks and fusions occur at exactly the same spot on each of the two strands. Therefore, genetic information is normally neither lost nor gained. However, because of this action, it is possible that genetic information which was originally on the individual's own paternal chromosome could break off and become attached to the individual's own maternal chromosome and vice versa. This phenomenon of exchange is known as *cross-over* or recombination and is a normal genetic event.

From a purely mechanical point of view, loci that are far apart on the chromosome have a greater chance of crossing-over than those that are close together. Therefore, such recombinations take place much more frequently. By counting gene combinations attributable to the gametes (sperm or ova) in offspring of infor-

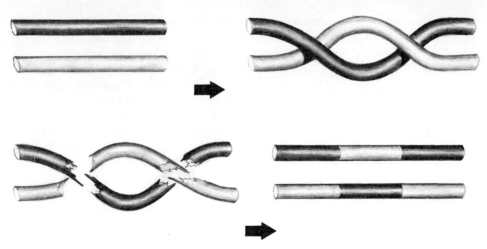

Fig. 1. A diagrammatic representation of the events resulting in the recombination of maternal and paternal genetic material during the formation of new gametes. The dark bar represents a portion of the paternal chromosome. The light bar represents a portion of chromosome originating from the mother. The two strands twist, break, and rejoin to form a totally new strand carrying some genetic material from each original parent.

mative families, one can calculate the frequency of cross-over between various loci. This frequency is known as the recombination fraction or cross-over frequency and is used by geneticists as a measure of the genetic distance between loci. The percent frequency is expressed in units known as centi-Morgans (cM), named after Thomas Hunt Morgan, the famous geneticist. A recombination frequency of 1% is equal to 1 cM of genetic distance between loci. Using this type of information, one can ascertain the spacial relationship of one locus to another and thereby effectively map the chromosome.

Loci that are so close together that recombination occurs less than 50% of the time are said to be linked. By definition a blood group system is composed of a series of alloantigenic red cell markers that are controlled by either a single locus or a series of linked loci that are independent (nonlinked) of any other blood group system. To be independent, i.e., segregate separately in families, the loci have to be either on a different pair of chromosomes or far enough apart on the same pair of chromosomes to allow for a 50% or greater frequency of recombination. If two loci are not linked but are found on the same pair of chromosomes, they are said to be *syntenic.*

To illustrate these points, take the two hypothetic loci A and B, each of which has its own series of alleles, such that *a, b, c,* and *d* are alleles at the A locus and *q, r, s,* and *t* are alleles at the B locus. (Note that symbols indicating genes are always in italics. Symbols for gene products are in roman type.)

When the inheritance of these alleles is examined in families, the following pattern will be observed if A and B loci are independent (not linked).

LOCI: A   B

$$\text{Alleles:} \begin{cases} a & q \\ b & r \\ c & s \\ d & t \end{cases}$$

NONLINKED LOCI

Parents: (A) a/b (B) q/r × (A) c/d (B) s,t

Possible gametes:

a,q	c,s
b,r	d,t
a,r	c,t
b,q	d,s

Offspring:

1/16 ac,qs	1/16 ad,qt	1/16 ac,qt	1/16 ad,qs
1/16 bc,rs	1/16 bd,rt	1/16 bc,rt	1/16 bd,rs
1/16 ac,rs	1/16 ad,rt	1/16 ac,rt	1/16 ad,rs
1/16 bc,qs	1/16 bd,qt	1/16 bc,qt	1/16 bd,qs

Therefore, if the A and B loci are not linked each offspring can be one of sixteen different combinations. This is in compliance with Mendel's law of independent assortment.

The situation is different if A and B are linked. For example:

LINKED LOCI

Parents: (AB) aq,br × (AB) cs/dt

Possible gametes:

aq	cs
br	dt

Offspring:

¼ aq/cs	¼ aq/dt
¼ br/cs	¼ br/dt

Thus, barring recombinations, which occur between linked loci with a frequency of less than 50%, each offspring can be only one of four different combinations.

The families that are most informative with respect to linkage and recombination are those in which one parent is heterozygous for both factors, while the other parent is homozygous for both. Such families make it possible to discern linkage with fewer offspring. In genetic experiments with plants and animals one can arrange such matings by performing a backcross, i.e., mating a heterozygous offspring back to one of its homozygous parents. Since two loci are involved and the parents must be homozygous for both, it is called a double backcross. In the study of human genetics, however, there are ethical and moral constraints against such a practice and the investigator must rely on the experiments of nature to provide the necessary material. Usually large numbers of families are studied and the results combined to establish linkage, using a method of analysis such as the Lod Score devised by Morton.[1]

Linkage and nonlinkage in double backcross families are shown by the following:

	LINKAGE		**NONLINKAGE**	
Parents:	*aq*	*cs*	*aq*	*cs*
	br ×	*cs*	*br* ×	*cs*
Gametes:	*aq* *cs*		*a,q* *c,s*	
	br		*b,r*	
Offspring:	½ *aq/cs*		¼ *a/c, q/s*	
	½ *br/cs*		¼ *b/c, r/s*	
			¼ *a/c, r/s*	
			¼ *b/c, q/s*	

When recombination occurs between the alleles of linked loci, the expected genotypes of the progeny will be the same as if there were no linkage; however, the frequency of the recombined types will be much lower than if the loci were independent. Therefore, in the example of linkage just shown, two additional parental gametes could result from recombination.

$$\text{Normal} \left\{ \begin{array}{ll} aq & cs \\ br & \end{array} \right.$$

$$\text{Gametes:} \quad \text{Recombined} \left\{ \begin{array}{l} ar \\ bq \end{array} \right.$$

Offspring: *aq/cs*
br/cs
(ar)/cs
(bq)/cs

All four types of progeny could be expected, but if the loci are linked the occurrence of the recombined gametes would be less than 50%. Thus the proportion of offspring bearing these gametes would not be as great as the one-fourth proportion of progeny that would be expected if the loci were independent.

Studies of linkage are an essential part of genetic investigations, but a clear distinction must be made between this phenomenon in its present sense and another phenomenon referred to as association. Linkage is a very precise genetic term that states unequivocally that two different and identifiable inherited traits are controlled by the same genetic units, and are found in a close and measurable proximity to one another on a single chromosome as defined by the frequency of recombination. This state can be deduced only from the study of informative families. Association, on the other hand, is a statistical term indicating that two measurable traits often accompany each other with some predictable probability that is greater than that which might be expected from chance alone. That two characteristics are associated with each other is an observable fact that provides no evidence for cause and effect and certainly no evidence for genetic linkage.

Crossing over and recombination of chromosomes is an entirely random event. Since this is the case, on a population level one would expect the assortment of alleles from separate but linked loci to be completely random. Again, take for example the two linked loci A and B with their allelic series:

$$\text{LOCUS:} \quad \textbf{A} \quad \textbf{B}$$

$$\text{Alleles:} \begin{cases} a & q \\ b & r \\ c & s \\ d & t \end{cases}$$

At genetic equilibrium one would expect the chromosomal combinations (haplotypes) aq, ar, as, at, bq, br, bs, bt, cq, cr, cs, ct, dq, dr, ds, and dt to occur in the populations being studied with a frequency that is equal to the product of the gene frequencies of the two alleles in that population. Stated another way, this means that every allele of the A locus has an equal chance of occurring on the same chromosome with every allele of the B locus and vice versa, constrained only by the frequency with which each occurs in the population under study.

In some cases associated with blood grouping, however, it might be discovered that certain combinations of alleles from the two loci predominate while the other combinations are rarely encountered. When this occurs, the alleles are said to exhibit linkage disequilibrium, which means that two genetically linked traits have failed to reach a state of equilibrium in the population by means of normal recombination. This could be due to a preferential lack of recombination because of selective advantage derived from the status quo or some other as yet unexplained biologic phenomenon.

The extent of linkage disequilibrium between two alleles at two closely linked loci can be measured. It is expressed as the difference between the observed and the randomly expected frequencies of the combination in the population. The difference, called delta (Δ), is a measure of this type of gametic association.

Phenotype expression need not be the result of single gene action. Sometimes the presence of another allele either on the same chromosome or on any other chromosome can influence the phenotypic expression of the allele whose gene product is being considered. This is referred to as *epistasis* and has considerable importance in the understanding of the genetics of blood group antigens.

In the days surrounding the early discovery of the blood group antigens, it was believed that each antigen was the product of the action of one gene. This was the concept of one gene–one antigen. It seemed to be a valid assumption at the time since little was known about the biochemical composition of the various antigens and even less about how genetic information was translated into immunologically functional structures.

The elucidation of the biochemistry of a number of the blood group antigens coupled with a firmer understanding of molecular genetics has altered this original concept considerably. It is now clear that blood group antigens whose specificity is an attribute of protein structures are coded for directly by appropriate genetic information, since genetic DNA has the ability to dictate the amino acid sequence and therefore the final configuration of protein molecules. On the other hand, blood group antigens that possess polysaccharide antigenic determinants are coded for indirectly. The genetic information directs the production of proteins that are highly specific enzymes, usually glycosyl transferases, which then act on appropriate carbohydrate substrates to construct the polysaccharide determinant itself. This implies the existence of at least one additional set of genes that code for the production of enzymes required for the assembly of the carbohydrate substrate. Several well-known and highly characterized blood group systems offer ample evidence that the final expression of polysaccharide antigenic determinants on the red cells' surface may involve the products of not only several structural genes but ones that may be at several independent loci. Further, on occasion even the production of protein antigens may be effected by epistatic modifier genes. Therefore, the old adage that one gene equals one antigen is no longer tenable in every case.

This fact must be considered when one is studying the genetics of the various blood group systems, since the phenotypic expression of the detectable gene products may be affected by genes at a number of other loci. A classic example of this type of interaction is illustrated by the Bombay phenotype of the ABO blood group system, which will be described in detail later. In this case the Bombay individuals do not exhibit the products of their ABO genes because, by virtue of their *hh* genotype at another locus, they are lacking the basic H precursor substance from which these antigens are made.

MATHEMATICAL AND STATISTICAL CONSIDERATIONS

Blood group systems, since they follow Mendelian laws, are established by family studies coupled with statistical tests of significance. Two of the laws of Mendel are especially appropriate to this discussion. The first is the law of segregation, which states that two alleles of a diploid individual segregate at meiosis with each allele going to a separate germ cell: the second is the law of independent assortment, which states that alleles at unlinked loci assort into the gametes independently of each other. These laws were derived from an observation of the relative proportion of the types of offspring obtained from various types of parental matings. The most basic observation was that the offspring of two parents, each of whom is heterozygous for a dominant trait, will be distributed phenotypically in a ratio of 3:1—three of the offspring will display the dominant trait while one will not. Extending this further, of the three dominant offspring, one will be homozygous for the dominant trait and two will be heterozygous. The remaining offspring not displaying the dominant trait must be homozygous for the recessive characteristic. This gives a genotype ratio of 1:2:1.

The mathematical and statistical considerations that pertain to genetic studies center about two questions. First, do the relative proportions of offspring from certain matings fall into the expected Mendelian ratios? Second, since there is error associated with all investigative procedures resulting from technical problems, sampling, and variations, the ratios actually observed may not correspond exactly to those predicted by the laws. Therefore, what is the probability that the results obtained from such studies are not merely due to chance, thereby invalidating any conclusions regarding concordance with Mendelian segregation?

To fully appreciate the Mendelian ratios and their derivation, it is worthwhile to consider some theoretical models of inheritance. Most terminal blood group genes exhibit neither dominance nor recessiveness and are fully expressed in spite of homozygosity of heterozygosity. This greatly simplifies the understanding of their inheritance, since in the majority of instances only the hereditary patterns to be discussed in the following section need be considered.

The very simplest model of this type of inheritance is one in which there are two factors, A and B, controlled by a single locus and so distributed that one parent has one factor and the other parent the second factor. All of the offspring from this mating will have both factors if the parents are both homozygous, which can be assumed to be the case when neither dominance nor recessiveness has to be considered. This can be illustrated by the following diagram:

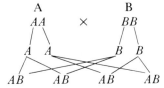

The same mating can be expressed in a tabular form using the Punnet Square. Here, the gametes of one parent are entered at the side, those of the other parent across the top. The combinations represent the results of random combination, which occurs at fertilization. (Effectively this is the same as algebraic multiplication.)

Paternal gametes

		A	*A*
Maternal gametes	*B*	*AB*	*AB*
	B	*AB*	*AB*

In the second model one of the parents carries both of the factors, A and B, and the other only one of them, A. Again, without considering dominance we can assume that one parent is heterozygous *AB* and the other homozygous *AA*. In this event one half of all the offspring will carry the same factor as the parent who is homozygous and the remaining half will be heterozygous and display both the A and the B factor.

The type of mating can be illustrated as follows:

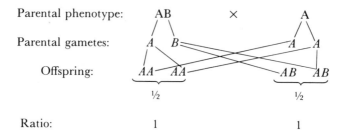

or in tabular form:

Paternal gametes

		A	*A*
Maternal gametes	*A*	*AA*	*AA*
	B	*AB*	*AB*

Finally, if each of the parents has both factors A and B, one fourth of the offspring will have only factor A, one fourth will have only factor B, and one half will have both factors A and B. Again by way of illustration:

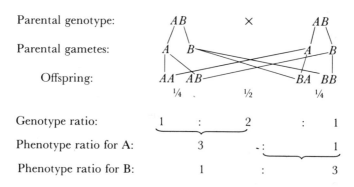

or in tabular form:

Paternal gametes

		A	*B*
Maternal gametes	*A*	*AA*	*AB*
	B	*BA*	*BB*

It should be pointed out that the two individuals AB and BA are identical genotypically and phenotypically with respect to the A and B factors in that both individuals have each of them. The only difference between them is the parental source of the particular factor. In the above example the offspring *AB* received the *A* from the father and the *B* from the mother while the *BA* individual received the *B* from the father and the *A* from the mother.

Variation within species results from gene changes. Such natural gene change or mutation, which ultimately gives rise to allelism, first occurs in one individual member of a species. Through the process of breeding over a very long period of time, the new allele is distributed throughout the population as a whole. Therefore not all alleles at a given locus are present in the same frequency. The percentage of all the genes for a particular trait that are of one kind is referred to as the *gene frequency*. The sum of all the gene frequencies for a given trait must always be 100% or 1.000. At any given point in time one would expect that every gene would have a specific gene frequency in the population that is in some way related to the efficiency with which it is spread. In humans the appearance of new alleles is a rare event since the mutation rate is very slow. Nevertheless, given long periods of time, differences in the gene frequencies of blood group alleles will occur among different populations. As a matter of fact an inordinately high gene frequency of one allele and a low gene frequency of another allele can frequently be associated with particular populations, races, or ethnic groups. For this reason many of the blood group antigens are useful as potent anthropologic markers.

In addition, excessive imbalance in the gene frequencies of certain alleles among various populations provides some interesting genetic problems. For example, it is possible that alleles with very low gene frequencies may be the result of mutations that occurred relatively recently. On the other hand, the high frequency alleles may have some advantage and are in the process of driving out the low frequency alleles.

Any population in which random mating occurs, barring such events as geographic migration, excessive inbreeding, or external catastrophic events, and if neither of the allelic conditions has any survival advantage nor is breeded for or against, will reach an equilibrium in which the gene frequencies will not change.

This condition, referred to as the Hardy-Weinberg equilibrium, can be appreciated best by understanding its derivation. Although this is detailed in a number of texts on general genetics, one of the clearest descriptions was given by Hackel.[2] The following explanation is adapted from that presentation.*

The simple mechanics of the monohybrid cross shown in Table 1, when considered for an entire population, lead to some interesting concepts about the population, and have been useful in elucidating the nature of a number of blood group systems.

In terms of individuals, this is simple enough. But when one is dealing with populations, a few other factors must be considered. If, of course, the population in question consists entirely of individuals having the same genotype and it is homozygous, there is no problem, since any offspring produced in this population will be of the same genotype as the parents. But if the population is not homozygous, the matter is not so simple.

---

* With permission of the author and the American Association of Blood Banks.

TABLE 1. MONOHYBRID CROSS

Parents:	*AA*	× ↓	*aa*
F_1 hybrids:	*Aa*	× ↓	*Aa*
F_2:	½ *AA* + ½ *Aa* + ¼ *aa*		

To make Table 1 applicable to populations rather than individuals, a theoretical model can be constructed based on several assumptions.

Let us assume a certain population to be made up of all *AA* people and another population entirely of *aa* people. Let them be of equal size and mix to form a new population. Let us assume that they are mating at random and the trait under consideration is not involved at all in mate selection, it does not confer any survival advantage or disadvantage on the individuals, and that this is a monogamous society and all mating pairs have the same number of offspring. In this new population four kinds of matings are possible, and on a probability basis, each of them would be expected with equal frequency. The details are shown in Table 2, and represent the concepts of Table 1 modified to apply to populations.

Thus the first new generation of the randomly mating theoretical population would consist of three different kinds of individuals in a definite proportion—one fourth are *AA*, one half *Aa*, and one fourth *aa*. When these offspring begin reproducing, nine different matings are possible, and some would occur more frequently than others. These are shown in Table 3.

From the frequencies of these matings it is possible to compute the nature and frequency of the offspring expected in the next generation, as is shown in Table 4.

Table 4 shows that the ratio of genotypes in the F_2 generation is unchanged from the F_1 generation. From this it can be reasoned that the proportion of geno-

TABLE 2. F_1 GENERATIONS OF A THEORETICAL POPULATION

Frequency of Matings	Male	Mating ×	Female	→	Offspring F_1	Proportion of New Generation	
¼	*AA*		*AA*		*AA*	¼	
¼	*AA*		*aa*		*Aa*	¼	½
¼	*aa*		*AA*		*Aa*	¼	
¼	*aa*		*AA*		*aa*	¼	

TABLE 3. MATING OF F_1 AND FREQUENCY OF EACH

♂ \ ♀	¼ **AA**	½ **Aa**	¼ **aa**
¼ *AA*	1/16	⅛	1/16
½ *Aa*	⅛	¼	⅛
¼ *aa*	1/16	⅛	1/16

TABLE 4. F$_2$ GENERATION OF THEORETICAL POPULATION

Frequency	Mating	Offspring	Proportion of New Generation
$\frac{1}{16}$	AA × AA	AA	$\frac{1}{16}$ AA
$2(\frac{1}{8})$	AA × Aa	$\frac{1}{2}$ AA + $\frac{1}{2}$ Aa	$\frac{1}{8}$ AA + $\frac{1}{8}$ Aa
$2(\frac{1}{16})$	AA × aa	Aa	$\frac{1}{8}$ Aa
$\frac{1}{4}$	Aa × Aa	$\frac{1}{4}$ AA + $\frac{1}{2}$ Aa + $\frac{1}{4}$ aa	$\frac{1}{16}$ AA + $\frac{1}{8}$ Aa + $\frac{1}{16}$ aa
$2(\frac{1}{8})$	AA × aa	$\frac{1}{2}$ Aa + $\frac{1}{2}$ aa	$\frac{1}{8}$ Aa + $\frac{1}{8}$ aa
$\frac{1}{16}$	aa × aa	aa	$\frac{1}{16}$ aa

$AA = \frac{1}{16} + \frac{1}{8} + \frac{1}{16} = \frac{1}{4}$
$Aa = \frac{1}{8} + \frac{1}{8} + \frac{1}{8} + \frac{1}{8} = \frac{1}{2}$
$aa = \frac{1}{16} + \frac{1}{8} + \frac{1}{16} = \frac{1}{4}$

types will remain the same for all successive generations, provided that no changes occur in the system of mating and no new genes are introduced into this population. It is said to be in equilibrium. Other numerical examples could be provided, all of which would lead to the same conclusion—with a population in equilibrium and satisfying the conditions mentioned earlier, the genotype frequencies, once established, do not change.

It should be apparent that we are dealing here with functions of the gene frequency. For example, of all the genes for the trait under consideration in our population, what percentages are *A* and what are *a?* Clearly, whatever percentage of *A* genes may occur, the differences between that and 100% will be the percentage of *a* genes, since the two together comprise all of the genes of this particular trait.

In the example, there were equal numbers of *AA* and *aa* individuals at the start. The frequency of the gene *A* at the start was 50% and so was that of gene *a*. When equilibrium was reached, regardless of genotypes, these were still the respective frequencies for *A* and *a*. To generalize this, the symbol "p" can be used for the *AA* part of the population and "q" for *aa*. Since these make up the entire population, p + q = 1, and p is the gene frequency of *A* and q is the gene frequency of *a*. Substituting this notation, the different possible matings are shown in Table 5.

Note that since the mating *AA × aa* may occur in two different ways (*AA × aa* and *aa × AA*), each of these must be considered and a factor of 2 used for this type of mating.

Continuing with this random mating and allowing all types of mating to occur in their expected frequencies, the F$_2$ generation can be obtained. Table 6 shows the

TABLE 5. F$_1$ GENERATION OF GENERALIZED POPULATION

Matings	Frequency	Offspring AA	Aa	aa
AA × AA	$p \times p = p^2$	p^2:		
2(AA × aa)	$2(p \times q) = 2pq$		2pq	
aa × aa	$q \times q = q^2$			q^2
	Total = p^2: *AA* +		2pq: *Aa* +	q^2: *aa*

frequencies of these matings, the nature of offspring expected from each, and the results in the next generation. Beneath the table the various terms are summarized.

And again, frequencies remain unchanged!

This statement, $p^2 + 2pq + q^2 = 1$, which is known as the Hardy-Weinberg principle (equilibrium), can be applied to any population mating at random. p and q are the gene frequencies of the two alleles in the population and from their value we can compute the expected frequencies of the three genotypes. Conversely, having the frequency of just one homozygous genotype enables us to compute the value of the other two genotypes.

CHI-SQUARE STATISTICS

One of the most frequently referred-to tests in blood group work is the chi-square (χ^2) test. Although an in-depth discussion of the basic principles of this test is beyond the scope of this book, some bare essentials of how the test can be used are definitely indicated.

The chi-square test, as it is employed, can be considered as a statistical test of goodness of fit or of independence of two events. Goodness of fit simply means how well an observed distribution of events corresponds to the distribution of events expected from the scientific hypothesis.

For example, the basic principle given by the Hardy-Weinberg equilibrium stipulates that the genes of a two-allele system are distributed in a population according to the binomial distribution $p^2 + 2pq + q^2 = 1$, where 1 is the mathematical equivalent of 100%. The proportion of each of the expected genotypes in the two-allele system can be calculated by substituting the appropriate gene frequencies in the binomial. This is the expected value, "E." By testing the population, one

TABLE 6. F_2 GENERATION OF GENERALIZED POPULATION

Mating	Frequency	Offspring AA	Aa	aa
AA × AA	$p^2 \times p^2 = p^4$	p^4		
AA × Aa	$2(p^2 \times 2pq) = 4p^3q$	$2p^3q$ +	$2p^3q$	
AA × aa	$2(p^2 \times q^2) = 2p^2q^2$		$2p^2q^2$	
Aa × Aa	$2pq \times 2pq = 4p^2q^2$	p^2q^2 +	$2p^2q^2$ +	p^2q^2
Aa × aa	$2(2pq \times q^2) = 4pq^3$		$2pq^3$ +	$2pq^3$
aa × aa	$q^2 \times q^2 = q^4$			q^4

Summarizing
proportion of all offspring:

$(p^4 + 2p^3q + p^2q^2)$ **AA** $+ (2p^3q + 4p^2q^2 + 2pq^3)$ **Aa** $+ (p^2q^2$ $+ 2pq^3 + q^4)$ **aa** $= p^2 (p^2 + 2pq + q^2)$ **AA** $+ 2pq (p^2 + 2pq + q^2)$ **Aa** $+ q^2 (p^2 + 2pq + q^2)$ **aa** $= p^2 (p + q)^2$ **AA** $+ 2pq (p + q)^2$ **Aa** $+ p^2 (p + q)^2$ **aa**.

Since $p + q = 1$ then the expression can be further reduced to equal: p^2 **AA** $+ 2pq$ **Aa** $+ q^2$ **aa** $= 100\%$ *of offspring.*

can determine the actual proportion of each genotype. These are the observed values, "O." In view of experimental variation it is unlikely that the values obtained experimentally will match exactly those obtained by calculation. As a matter of fact, some investigators become highly suspicious if they do give an exact match! Therefore, some statistical inference will be required to determine how closely the observed values approach the ideal distribution. The chi-square test can be performed to see how well the distribution of observed values fits the distribution of values expected if they are distributed according to a binomial.

The formula for Chi-square is given as:

$$\chi^2 = \Sigma \frac{(0 - E)^2}{E}$$

In practice the quantity $\frac{(0 - E)^2}{E}$ is calculated for each of the points on the distribution, i.e., the p^2, the $2pq$ and the q^2. These are then added and the sum (Σ) is equal to χ^2.

A table of $\varkappa^2$ (Appendix 4) is then consulted to obtain a value of "p" or the probability that the differences obtained between the observed and expected values could be as great or greater than they are due to chance alone.[3] If the p value is high, 0.90 or greater, it indicates that differences as great or greater than those observed could be obtained purely by chance 90 times out of 100. Therefore it can be inferred that the differences obtained are most likely due only to chance or experimental variation and the hypothesis that the observed distribution is the equivalent of the expected binomial distribution is supported. Conversely, if the p value is lower than 0.05, the differences between observed and expected is too great to be attributed to chance and the hypothesis is not supported. The $\varkappa^2$ table is arranged according to degrees of freedom, df. In testing the goodness of fit to a binomial, one degree of freedom is lost as a result of the total and another from the estimation of the gene frequency from the population. Therefore, $df = n - 2$ where n equals the number of comparisons that went into the total $\varkappa^2$. Since a binomial contains three comparisons, $df = 3 - 2 = 1$.

Chi-square can also be used as a test of independence in what is known as a 2 × 2 contingency test. This technique is useful for ascertaining whether two antigens are associated with each other genetically or whether they are independent. It is also useful in the identification of antibodies when an exact match between the reactions of an antiserum and the occurrence of antigens among the cells of a test panel is not readily discernible because of technical problems, the presence of multiple antibodies, weak reactions, etc.

An example of the second instance is given to illustrate the mechanics of 2 × 2 comparisons. A sample of patient's serum believed to contain antibodies may be tested against a panel of red cells from twenty different people whose blood groups are known. The serum reacts with several of the twenty cells, leading one to ask the question, what is the most likely specificity of the antibody?

To obtain an idea of the answer to this question, a 2 × 2 table can be constructed and the chi-square test performed. In this type of test, if two events being compared are independent (in this case the occurrence of a certain antigen on some of the cells and the positive reaction of the unknown antibody with this group of the cells), x^2 value will be low. On the other hand, if the two events are *not* independent the x^2 value will be high. Stated another way, when the x^2 is low the probability of independence is high, and when the x^2 is high the probability of independence is low. As a matter of fact, if this probability is low enough, 0.01–0.001 or less, there is a fairly good chance that the events are not only not independent but actually totally dependent on each other. When the reactions of an unknown serum are compared with the antigens in a panel, this dependence is usually one of cause and effect and in the most obvious cases indicates that the antibody may be indeed directed toward that particular antigenic specificity. An example of this is given below:

Reaction of anti-unknown

		+	−	
Distribution of antigen x	+	a	b	a + b
	−	c	d	c + d
		a + c	b + d	n

The χ^2 is computed according to the formula where n = a + b + c + d

$$\frac{(ad - cb)^2 n}{(a + b)(c + d)(a + c)(b + d)} = \chi^2$$

Substituting real numbers:

	+	−	
+	6	0	6
−	1	13	14
	7	13	20

$$\frac{(6 \cdot 13 - 1.0)^2 \, 20}{6 \cdot 14 \cdot 7 \cdot 13} = \chi^2$$
$$\chi^2 = 15.9$$

According to the table of the chi-square distribution for 1 df (2 × 2 contingency tables have 1 df), this x^2 value corresponds to a p of less than 0.0005. Therefore, the occurrence of the antigen in the panel and the reaction of the unknown antibody are not independent events. It is probable that the antibody in question is anti-X and the false positive reaction observed with one of the cells may be due to the presence of a second antibody or to some technical or clerical error.

The same procedure may be used to ascertain the likelihood of two sera containing antibodies of the same specificity. In such an investigation the two sera are tested simultaneously against a large panel of random cells. The positive and negative reactions of each are then compared in a 2 × 2 contingency test. Very low p values are a good indicator that antibodies are identical, but of course this must be confirmed by further serologic tests such as absorption.

As stated previously, the 2 × 2 contingency chi-square is useful as an indicator of the genetic relationship of two antigens. For example, if two antigens tend to occur together in the population, as evidenced from a high chi-square (lack of independence) in this type of comparison, it is possible that they may be the product of linked or perhaps syntenic loci. On the other hand, two antigens may give a high chi-square; however, an examination of the 2 × 2 table itself reveals that the cross product, ad is much smaller than the cross product, bc. In other words, most of the time the first antigen is present only when the second one is absent and vice versa. Such a finding indicates a negative association between the two antigens and could indicate that they are the products of allelic genes. In either case, these are merely indicators and specific genetic tests for either linkage or allelism must be performed for confirmation.

The chi-square for a 2 × 2 table can be calculated in the manner just described only in those cases when n, i.e., the total number of comparisons, is 10 or greater. One of the reasons for attaching this condition is that when the two variables being compared are identical, chi-square = n. [In this case b = 0 and c = 0, therefore the cross product b × c = 0, and since the remaining cross product $(a × d)^2$ equals the product of the marginal totals, (a + 0) (0 + d) (a + 0) (0 +d), these terms cancel out, leaving n = x^2.] For 1 df, two variables known to be identical when compared in five instances would give a probability greater than 0.02. This, of course, would lead to a false assumption.

Therefore, when fewer than ten comparisons are made, the probability of chance must be calculated directly using Fisher's exact test. This is done in the following manner. Given a 2 × 2 table:

		x		
		+	−	
y	+	a	b	a + b
	−	c	d	c + d
		a + c	b + d	n

The formula for the exact test is:

$$p = \frac{(a + b)\,!\,(c + d)\,!\,(a + c)\,!\,(b + d)\,!}{n\,!\,a\,!\,b\,!\,c\,!\,d\,!}$$

Two conditions are placed on the use of this test: 1. n must be less than 20, and 2. one of the cells, a, b, c, or d, must be equal to zero. If one of the cells is not zero the following procedure must be used. Given the table:

		x +	x −	
y	+	3	9	12
y	−	6	2	8
		9	11	20

$$p_1 = \frac{(12\,!)\,(8\,!)\,(9\,!)\,(11\,!)}{(20\,!)\,(3\,!)\,(9\,!)\,(6\,!)\,(2\,!)} = 0.0367$$

The table is then rearranged by lowering the lowest value by one but retaining the same marginal totals:

		x +	x −	
y	+	2	10	12
y	−	7	1	8
		9	11	20

$$p_2 = \frac{(12\,!)\,(8\,!)\,(9\,!)\,(11\,!)}{(20\,!)\,(2\,!)\,(10\,!)\,(7\,!)\,(1\,!)} = 0.0031$$

The same procedure must be repeated until the smallest value becomes zero. Thus another rearrangement gives:

	+	−	
+	1	11	12
−	8	0	8
	9	11	20

$$p_3 = \frac{(12\,!)\,(8\,!)\,(9\,!)\,(11\,!)}{(20\,!)\,(1\,!)\,(11\,!)\,(8\,!)\,(0\,!)} = 0.001$$

The total probability (Pt) that the extent of discrepancies obtained between x and y is as great or greater due to chance is $Pt = p_1 + p_2 + p_3 = 0.0367 + 0.0031 + 0.001 = 0.0399$. The interpretation of this p value is the same as that attached to the p value obtained from the standard chi-square test.

ELUCIDATION OF BLOOD GROUP SYSTEMS

The principles discussed in the previous sections are essential in understanding the concepts used in the elucidation of a blood group system. If for example, a new blood group antigen is discovered, it is possible to assign a hypothetical gene symbol "A" to the new antigen and to test a large population with the antisera defining this antigen. The positives would be either A^2 or Aa, but the negatives would all be assigned to the a^2 class. Using this assumption one can calculate the gene frequency of the a allele from the equation for the binomial. This is equal to the square root of the homozygous state of a. Then, by employing the equation, one can calculate the gene frequency of a.

Using these data, one can now calculate the relative proportion of the three hypothetic genotypes in the populations as well as the frequency of the expected matings between genotypes and the frequency of the various progeny. Family studies can be carried out to obtain the actual values for the frequencies, which are then compared with the calculated values, using a test of statistical significance.

A sample computation involving the genesis of a hypothetical blood group system and employing the principles described follows.

Step 1. Discovery of a monospecific antiserum detecting a new blood group antigen called "Z." Therefore, the antibody becomes anti-Z.

Step 2. Test a large population with anti-Z to obtain two groups:

Group 1	Z+	99 =	8.94% =	0.0894
Group 2	Z−	1,009 =	91.06% =	0.9106
	Total	1,108	100.00%	1.0000

When a new blood group antigen is discovered, it is assumed to be the result of genetic information. Thus the presence of such an antigen requires that the appropriate gene also be present. Therefore those individuals bearing the Z antigen must have at least one Z gene to have produced the antigen. They may also be homozygous for this gene:

$$\left.\begin{array}{l} ZZ \\ Zz \end{array}\right\} \text{ Z positive}$$

It follows, then, that those persons negative for the antigen Z must lack the Z gene and have the genotype zz.

Step 3. Calculate the gene frequency of Z, which is the square root of the frequency of the homozygous state, by employing the following reasoning:

a. Assuming there are two genes, Z and z, then:
$Zz \times Zz$ mating results in offspring ZZ, Zz, zZ, zz.

b. Mathematically this can be represented as a binomial:
$Z^2 + 2Zz + z^2 = 1.000$.

c. Since the $Z-$ individuals from the population can be assumed to have the genotype zz, the gene frequency of this hypothetic allele can be calculated directly:
Gene frequency of $z = \sqrt{0.9106} = 0.9543$.

d. Since the combined frequency of the two genes in the population is equal to 1.000, the gene frequency of Z can be obtained by subtraction:
Gene frequency of $Z = 1 - z = 1 - 0.9543 = 0.0457$.

e. As a proof:
$(0.0457)^2 + 2(0.0457)(0.9543) + (0.9543)^2 = 0.9999$ or 1.000.

Step 4. Using the gene frequencies one can calculate the expected genotype frequencies in the population:

$$\begin{aligned}
ZZ &= (0.0457)(0.0457) = 0.0021 = 0.21\% \\
Zz &= 2(0.0457)(0.9107) = 0.0872 = 8.72\% \\
zz &= 0.9107 = 0.9107 = 91.07\%
\end{aligned}$$

Step 5. Based on the hypothetical genotype frequencies in the population, the frequency of matings and offspring can be calculated: e.g., the frequency with which $Z+ \times Z+$ mating occurs is equal to:

MATINGS

1. $ZZ \times ZZ = (0.0021)(0.0021) = 0.0000044$
2. $ZZ \times Zz = 2(0.0021)(0.0872) = 0.0003632$
3. $Zz \times Zz = (0.0872)(0.0872) = 0.0076038$

Total $Z+ \times Z+$ $= 0.0079714$

Thus, 0.0079714 represents the proportion of all matings which will be $Z+ \times Z+$.

The frequency of offspring from each genotype of $Z+ \times Z+$ mating is equal to:

CHILDREN

	ZZ	*Zz*	*zz*
From 1. All ZZ	= 0.0000044	0	0
From 2. ½ZZ, ½ZZ	= 0.0001832	0.0001832	0
From 3. ¼ZZ, ½ZZ, ¼ZZ	= 0.0019009	0.0038019	0.0019009
Total	0.0020841	0.0039851	0.0019009

The proportion of all of the children that result from all types of $Z+ \times Z+$ matings is: $0.0020841 + 0.0039851 + 0.0019009 = .0079714$.

Of these $\dfrac{0.0019009}{0.0079714} = 0.2385$ will be $Z-$ children and $\dfrac{0.0020841 + 0.0039851}{0.0079714} +$ 0.7615 will be $Z+$ children.

Step 6. Using the new reagent (anti-Z), a large number of families is tested. The expected distribution is calculated and compared with the observed:

| | MATINGS | | CHILDREN | | | |
| | | | Z+ | | Z− | |
Type	Ob-served	Ex-pected	Ob-served	Ex-pected	Ob-served	Ex-pected
Z+ × Z+	4	2.68	7	8.39	4	2.62
Z+ × Z−	57	54.63	69	69.08	66	65.92
Z− × Z−	275	278.67	0	0.00	597	597.00

The expected values are calculated according to Step 5, using the actual number in the family study, e.g., the expected number of Z+ × Z+ matings in the sample of 336 families tested should be: 336 (0.0079714) = 2.68.

Of such matings there were eleven children; thus the number of Z− among them was expected to be 11 (0.2385) = 2.62.

Step 7. Each of the observed and expected values over 10 are then subjected to the chi-square test.

$$\chi^2 = \frac{(\text{observed} - \text{expected})^2}{\text{expected}}$$

The chi-square values obtained for each of the comparisons are added. The probability that the difference obtained between the observed and expected values could be as great or greater than those obtained due to chance alone is taken from a table of chi-square values.

If the likelihood (probability) of the difference between the observed and expected values being due to chance is sufficiently great (90 in 100 or 999 in 1,000), then the original hypothesis of a system is tentatively accepted.

Step 8. Confirmation results from the discovery of the second antibody, anti-z, which detects the products of the postulated allele z.

THE ABO SYSTEM

The most important human blood groups belong to the ABO system. This system is frequently referred to as the Major Blood Group System since it allows a primary classification of all humans into one of four groups: A, B, O, and AB. In addition, the system is of paramount importance in clinical blood transfusion. It was discovered by Landsteiner in 1900: a translation of his original paper is reprinted in the appendix.

Like all of the other blood group systems, the classification is based on the occurrence of genetically controlled antigenic characteristics present on the surface of erythrocytes that are discernible with specific antibodies. Antigenic characteristics such as these, which distinguish one member of a species from another member of the same species, are referred to as *alloantigens*.

In his experiments, Landsteiner collected blood samples from five of his associates and from himself. The blood was allowed to clot and the sera separated from the red cells. He then mixed each serum with each of the individual cell suspensions and looked for a reaction. He saw that some of the suspensions were agglutinated by the sera of certain individuals and others were not. The results of his experiment are shown in Table 7. Landsteiner concluded that these reactions were attributable to the presence or absence of two agglutinable antigens, A and B, on the surface of the red blood cells. Dr. Ple. and Zar. possessed the A antigen and, therefore, belonged to blood group A, while Dr. Sturl. and Dr. Erd. possessed the B antigen, placing them in blood group B. Dr. St. and Landsteiner himself had neither of these antigens, and therefore were classified as null or group O.

Since none of these experimental subjects had been previously immunized, Landsteiner further concluded that all people must have natural antibodies (isoagglutinins) in their sera directed against the antigen that is absent from their own cells. Therefore, one would expect people belonging to group A to have anti-B (β) antibodies in their sera, those belonging to group B to have anti-A (α) in their sera, and those belonging to group O to possess both anti-A and anti-B (α, β). This relationship was further borne out by the investigations of two of his associates, von Decastello and Sturli who, in 1902, found a person who possessed both the A and B antigens on his red cells. This person was, therefore, classified as belonging to the rare blood group AB. As expected, neither anti-A nor anti-B could be detected in his serum. Landsteiner was lucky in his discovery, in that the antigens of this blood group system are so readily definable with antibodies that are present in the sera of all individuals, without the benefit of apparent antigenic stimulus.

In the routine laboratory, specially prepared and commercially available blood-grouping sera containing either anti-A or anti-B are used to identify the four groups. Such sera will agglutinate the cells containing the corresponding antigens according to the scheme shown in Table 8. It has been repeatedly demonstrated that the isoagglutinins occur with precise regularity in the sera of all adult individu-

TABLE 7. THE RESULTS OF LANDSTEINER'S EXPERIMENT ON THE HUMAN BLOOD GROUPS

| Sera | Cells | | | | | | Antibody |
	Dr. St.	Dr. Ple.	Dr. Sturl.	Dr. Erd.	Zar.	Landst.	
Dr. St.	−	+	+	+	+	−	α and β
Dr. Ple.	−	−	+	+	−	−	β
Dr. Sturl.	−	+	−	−	+	−	α
Dr. Erd.	−	+	−	−	+	−	α
Zar	−	−	+	+	−	−	β
Landst.	−	+	+	+	+	−	α and β
Antigen	O	A	B	B	A	O	

TABLE 8. THE REACTIONS OF THE CELLS AND THE SERA
BELONGING TO THE MEMBERS OF THE FOUR ABO
BLOOD GROUPS

Blood Group	RBC Tested with		Serum Tested with	
	Anti-A	Anti-B	A-Cells	B-Cells
A	+	−	−	+
B	−	+	+	−
O	−	−	+	+
AB	+	+	−	−

als in association with these groups. Therefore, their demonstration is mandatory for the definitive classification.

Those people belonging to blood group O possess neither the A nor the B antigens. However, their cells do possess a large amount of an antigen called H. The H antigen is an important antigen since it is the basic ground substance from which the A and B antigens are derived, as shown by its chemical structure.

These alloantigenic characteristics are well-developed structures even in a thirty-seven-day-old fetus and remain prominent throughout a person's lifetime. The required alloantibodies (previously called isoagglutinins), however, are not found at birth for two major reasons. First, the newborn human's immune system is still too immature at birth to form the appropriate antibodies, and second, the newborn has not yet been exposed to the appropriate normal bacteria containing the cross-reactive antigens against which these antibodies are found.

The A, B, and H antigens are present not only on the red cells, but exist in varying concentration in most of the other body tissues, with the exception of the brain and the spinal cord, as an intimate part of the cell wall. It was first believed that the cellular antigens in tissues as well as red cells were lipidlike materials, because they could be extracted with alcohol but not with water. Subsequent biochemical studies have shown that the antigens are complex and highly branched glycosphingolipids. The lipid portion of these molecules serves as an attachment to the red cell surface through the fluid mosaic of the membrane, while a branched glycoprotein is exposed above the surface and endows the molecule with its serologic specificity.

In addition to possessing these antigens on the surface of their red cells and other tissues, 78% of people possess soluble antigens in their body secretions with a specificity corresponding to their own individual ABO groups. These antigens are water-soluble glycoproteins. They can be detected in the saliva, urine, sweat, tears, gastric juice, bile, and even serum, but not in the cerebrospinal fluid. People whose body fluids contain blood group substances are known as *secretors*. The remaining 22 percent of the population whose A, B, or H blood group antigens are found only on the tissues are called *nonsecretors*. Although these people fail to secrete A, B, or H they do secrete a blood group antigen known as Le[a] or Lewis, which will be discussed later. The ability to transform soluble secretions into blood group antigens is a hereditary characteristic controlled by means of two allelomorphic genes, *Se* and *se*. The gene for secretion, *Se*, is dominant while its allele, *se*, is recessive. Therefore, individuals of genotype *SeSe* or *Sese* are secretors while those having a genotype *sese* are nonsecretors.

The secretor genes belong to a system that is genetically independent of ABO. However, they play a significant role in the complex chain of events that leads to the formation of the A, B, and H antigens.

Not all individuals belonging to blood group A or the blood group AB are alike since the A characteristic can be serologically divided into the subgroups A_1 and A_2. As early as 1911, von Dungern and Hirszfeld showed that when an anti-A serum from a group B individual was absorbed with group A red cells from a selected donor, not all of the anti-A was removed. The resultant serum still reacted with some but not all group A individuals, as shown in Table 9. The group A individuals who still reacted with the serum were called A_1, and the ones who failed to react were called A_2.

Therefore, there are two basic kinds of A antigen, A_1 and A_2. In addition, as shown by von Dungern's experiment, there are two kinds of anti-A antibody. One of these, anti-A_1 reacts only with A_1 cells, whereas the other, anti-A_{common}, reacts with all group A red cells, including the A_2 cells that must have been used for the absorption.

Thus, by the use of an unabsorbed anti-A serum and an anti-A_1 serum prepared by absorption with group A_2 cells, one can subdivide group A individuals into A_1 and A_2 and group AB individuals into A_1B and A_2B. This distinction, however, can only be made between the cells of adults, since the A_1 antigen does not attain its full in vitro serologic characteristics until after the first year of life.

Besides using reagents prepared by absorption, or those found in the sera of group A_2B individuals, one can distinguish group A_1 cells by means of specific phytohemagglutinins or lectins. Many of these compounds have been isolated from the seeds of leguminous plants. Lectins are not true antibodies but by chance have a chemical configuration complementary to polysaccharide blood group antigens and can cause specific clumping of red blood cells. A large number have been found that react with numerous antigenic determinants. An anti-A_1 lectin of this type, prepared from the seeds of *Dolichos bioflorus,* is commercially available.

An anti-A_2 serum cannot be prepared by absorbing an anti-A serum with A_1 cells, since the A_2 antigen does not exist as a separate entity. It is merely an A antigen devoid of an A_1 component. Nevertheless, the sera of certain A_1 and A_1B individuals may contain weak antibodies that will agglutinate A_2 cells and O cells. These agglutinins are in reality anti-H. The fact that these antibodies react more

**TABLE 9. AGGLUTINATION REACTIONS OF AN
ABSORBED ANTI-A SERUM**

| | Group B Serum | | |
| | | Absorbed with | |
Test Cells	Unabsorbed	A_1 Cells	A_2 Cells
A_1	++++	−	+++
A_2	++++	−	−

strongly with A_2 cells than with A_1 cells leads to the conclusion that A_2 cells contain H antigen in greater amounts than A_1 cells. This has been corroborated by studies with the anti-H lectins from both *Ulex europeus* and *Lotus tetragonolobus.*

From a routine clinical standpoint the subgroups of A are not considered. However, on occasion they may become important since the sera of a certain proportion of group A_2 individuals and an even greater proportion of group A_2B individuals contain a specific anti-A_1 agglutinin. Although these antibodies usually react only at low temperatures, they can cause cross-matching difficulties and clinical problems under the appropriate circumstances.

In addition to A_1 and A_2 a number of other less frequent and unusual subgroups of A have been described. These are summarized in Figure 2. By and large they are all characterized by being composed of ever-decreasing amounts of A and increasing amounts of H. None of these, however, has the distinction of carrying a distinctive specificity such as that found in A_1.

The various subgroups of A may also be found in combination with B. The *B* gene exerts a quenching effect on A, so that the A subgroups in AB individuals appear even weaker, giving fragile agglutinates, lower titration scores, and having less absorption power.

The A, B, and H antigens exist in two distinct forms—as glycoproteins in the secretions of secretors and as glycolipids in cell membranes. Over the years a great deal of biochemical data has been amassed on the structure and composition of these antigens, and it is evident that the polysaccharide portion of both is similar. There are two types of basic chains composed of four sugar residues—galactose, *n*-acetylglucosamine, galactose, *n*-acetylgalactosamine—that are bound to polypeptides (Fig. 3). Each of the antigenic specificities is caused by different terminal sugars attached to the basic chain; fucose for H, *n*-acetylgalactosamine for A, and galactose for B. The attachment is accomplished by means of highly specific glyco-

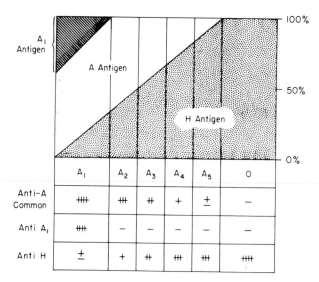

	A_1	A_2	A_3	A_4	A_5	0
Anti-A Common	+++	++	+	+	±	−
Anti A_1	+++	−	−	−	−	−
Anti H	±	+	++	+++	+++	+++

Fig. 2. The hypothetical quantitative distribution of A and H antigens within the various subgroups of A.

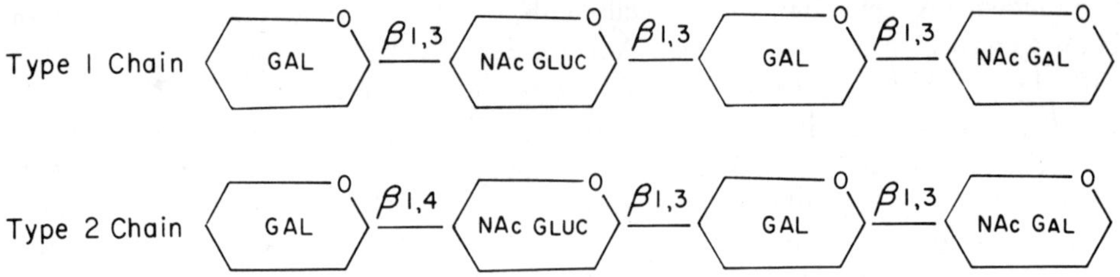

Fig. 3. The chemical structure of the two types of base chains forming the polysaccharide backbone of A, B, and H blood group substances. These chains exist in nature as branches composed of the type 1 and type 2 structures.

syl transferases that are formed through the action of the appropriate *A, B,* and *O* genes.

The two types of basic chain differ only in that the type 1 structure the terminal galactose is bound to *n*-acetylglucosamine through a $\beta 1,3$ linkage, whereas in type 2 the linkage is $\beta 1,4$. The type 1 and type 2 chains serve as precursor substances from which the A, B, and H antigens are formed.

Interestingly, the type 2 chain is identical with a polysaccharide structure found in the capsule of type XIV pneumococcus. As a matter of fact, the A, B, and H antigens of humans appear to be ubiquitous in nature. A variety of compounds bearing a very close serologic resemblance to these determinants have been found in many species of bacteria, particularly the gram-negative coliforms, in plants and animals. Among the animals, great apes and monkeys may have either A-like or B-like substances as alloantigenic characteristics. In addition, the gastric mucosa of hogs is an excellent source of A antigen while a fully reactive B preparation can be made from the same organ of the horse (see Chapter 9).

The ABO blood groups are inherited through a system containing three major allelic genes, *A, B,* and *O,* operative at a single genetic locus. It should be borne in mind that the *A* gene can be either an A_1 gene or an A_2 gene. The possible phenotypes and genotypes are shown in Table 10. The *A* and *B* genes are codominant and the *O* gene is an amorph, i.e., a gene that does not express itself phenotypically. One of the three possible genes is transmitted to an offspring by each of the two parents. They then combine to form one of two possible genotype combinations, giving rise to one of the four possible phenotypes discernible in the reactions with the standard anti-A and anti-B antisera. The expected offspring of various possible matings are given in Table 11 and the frequencies of the most common phenotypes are shown in Table 12.

One of the principal conclusions that follows from this scheme is that the mating of O to AB could never result in an AB offspring. However, several cases have been referred to by Race and Sanger[3] that clearly indicate the occasional occurrence of *A* and *B* alleles in the cis position, i.e., both present on the same chromosome. As the authors point out, this could be due to either recombination or a very infrequent *AB* allele.

It is not possible to distinguish the A or B phenotypes resulting from the genotypes *AA* or *BB* from those resulting from the genotypes *AO* or *BO* except by family

TABLE 10. GENOTYPES OF THE FOUR ABO GROUPS

ABO Group (Phenotype)	Genotypes
A	A/A, A/O
B	B/B, B/O
O	O/O
AB	A/B
A_1	A_1/A_1, A_1/A_2, A_1/A_3, A_1/A_4, A_1/A_5, A_1/O
A_2	A_2/A_2, A_2/A_3, A_2/A_4, A_2/A_5, A_2/O
A_3	A_3/A_3, A_3/A_4, A_3/A_5, A_3/O
A_4	A_4/A_4, A_4/A_5, A_4/O
A_5	A_5/A_5, A_5/O
A_1B	A_1/B
A_2B	A_2/B
A_3B	A_3/B
A_4B	A_4/B
A_5B	A_5/B

TABLE 11. GENOTYPES EXPECTED IN OFFSPRING RESULTING FROM VARIOUS MATINGS

Mating	Expected Offspring
$A/A \times A/A$	A/A
$A/A \times A/O$	A/A, A/O
$A/A \times B/B$	A/B
$A/A \times B/O$	A/B, A/O
$A/A \times A/B$	A/A, A/B
$A/A \times O/O$	A/O
$A/O \times A/O$	A/A, A/O, O/O
$A/O \times B/B$	A/B, B/O
$A/O \times B/O$	A/B, O/O, A/O, B/O
$A/O \times A/B$	A/A, A/B, A/O, B/O
$A/O \times O/O$	A/O, O/O
$B/B \times B/B$	B/B
$B/B \times B/O$	B/B, B/O
$B/B \times A/B$	A/B, B/B
$B/B \times O/O$	B/O
$B/O \times B/O$	B/B, B/O, O/O
$B/O \times A/B$	A/B, B/B, A/O, B/O
$B/O \times O/O$	B/O, O/O
$A/B \times A/B$	A/A, A/B, B/B
$A/B \times O/O$	A/O, B/O
$O/O \times O/O$	O/O

studies, since an anti-O capable of reacting with the supposed product of the O gene in single dose cannot be formed. In 1952, the Bombay phenotype referred to previously was described by Bhende et al.[4] Erythrocytes belonging to this phenotype were completely devoid of A, B, or H antigens, overtly resembling the blood group O (except for the lack of the H antigen).

TABLE 12. PHENOTYPE FREQUENCIES ABO

Phenotype	White (%)	Black (%)
O	45.58	49.09
A	40.63	27.66
A_1	29.00	19.60
A_2	8.90	6.80
B	10.07	19.90
AB	3.70	3.33

$A_1B : A_2B$ ratio = 3.71 A_1B : 1.00 A_2B

In a mating of Bombay (O) to A_1B, A_1B offspring resulted. As an explanation for the occurrence of this phenomenon, the brilliant geneticist Ceppellini[5] postulated the existence of inhibitor genes. These genes could, in some manner, control the expression of the antigens on the red cells' surface. Watkins and Morgan[6] proposed that a pair of genes, H and h, controlling the production of the H antigen and independent of the A, B, O genes, were responsible. A scheme showing the genetic pathways leading to the formation of these antigens is depicted in Figure 4.

According to this scheme, which has been substantiated with ample biochemical evidence, some precursor substance is first acted on by the H and h genes. H is dominant; therefore, individuals of HH or Hh genotype manufacture the H antigen. Those people whose genotype is hh cannot convert the precursor to H antigen. Next the A, B, O genes come into play. The dominant A and B genes act upon the H substance to produce either various amounts or various kinds of A or B depending

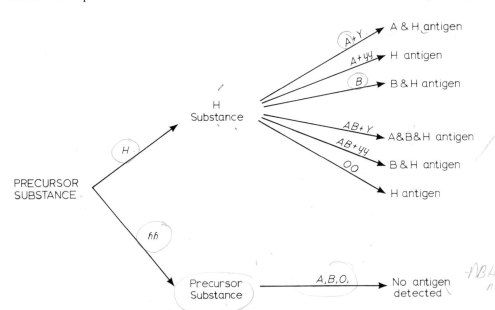

Fig. 4. Genetic pathway leading to the production of the A, B, and H antigens on the red blood cells. (*After Watkins and Morgan*[6] *and Ceppellini.*[5])

on whether the individual is A_1, A_2, A_3, or B_1, B_2, and so forth. The O gene is an amorph and effects no conversion, so that unaltered H antigen is passed on to the cells. Bombay individuals who are hh do not manufacture H antigen, so there is no substrate on which their A, B, or O genes can act. Therefore, their erythrocytes contain no discernible antigens even though they carry the appropriate terminal genes, which can be transmitted to their offspring. Because the Hh genes are transmitted independently of the A, B, O genes and h is recessive and is required to be present in double dose to exert its suppressor effect, frequently the offspring will possess a demonstrable antigen when none was present on one of the parent's cells. Thus the peculiar Bombay phenotype can be explained.

The general concept that alloantigens are genetically controlled characteristics, unalterable throughout the life of an individual, has become a well-accepted principle. A single system is composed of a group of antigenic determinants whose serologic specificity is controlled by genes that occur at either the same locus or closely associated loci on the same chromosome. Thus, the genes controlling a series of antigens of one blood group system are always inherited en bloc from a single parent, with genetic crossing-over occurring only infrequently.

The detectable antigen is a phenotypic expression of the genes of the blood group system. However, the phenotype can often be misleading since it is now apparent that the route by which the antigens are formed is not a direct one but can be influenced by many unrelated and unlinked genes at many loci.

There are some exceptions to these rules. For example, cases have been reported in which the A antigen of adult red cells has been considerably weakened or even lost altogether. Most of these apparent changes in blood groups have occurred in patients suffering from leukemia. Some authors feel that such a change could be the result of a somatic mutation, induced by the presence of a malignancy, but others believe it arises as a result of the treatment of the disease. In some cases of leukemia, during the course of a clinical remission the expression of antigenic strength returns to normal. Numerous theories can be postulated to explain these findings. It is quite possible that during the course of a severely debilitating disease, a lack of suitable substrate ensues. Thus, the appropriate antigens cannot be manufactured even if unmutated genes are available and functioning. Furthermore, the possibility cannot be ignored that the disease has produced abnormal serum or cell factors that adversely affect the test systems.

THE ABO ALLOANTIBODIES

The anti-A and anti-B antibodies, still frequently referred to as *isoagglutinins,* occur with precise regularity in the sera of all individuals. Therefore their presence or absence must be ascertained for the definitive establishment of the groups. In most cases, the absence of an expected agglutinin or the presence of an extra agglutinin is the first indication of some abnormality with either the inheritance or the expression of the A, B, or H antigens. For example, the absence of an anti-A agglutinin in the serum of a person whose red cells do not react with the standard anti-A and anti-B blood-grouping reagents (thereby appearing to be blood group O) is fairly strong evidence that the person may belong to some weak form of blood group A. Similarly, the appearance of an anti-H antibody in the serum of a group O person is a clue to the existence of the rare Bombay phenotype.

In addition to anti-A and anti-B the sera of approximately 2% of A_2 individuals and 26% of A_2B individuals contain anti-A_1 antibodies. Anti-A_1 may also be found in the sera of members of some of the other A subgroups, but not with any degree of regularity. Anti-H occurs in the sera of Bombay individuals and may occasionally be found in the sera of some A_1 and A_1B individuals.

Because the alloantibodies in this system occur with such predictable regularity in all individuals without any apparent overt antigenic stimulation, they have been referred to as naturally occurring. They normally appear in the serum three to six months after birth and remain throughout life. One may find considerable variation in the amount of these antibodies present in the serum of a person during his or her life-span. At first they are present in low titer, which gradually increases to a peak shortly after adolescence. The titer remains fairly constant through middle age, then begins to subside, reaching a low during senescence. These are average titers, however, and day-to-day as well as seasonal variation about any mean titer can be observed, depending to a certain extent on the person's general state of health.

The sera of newborn infants are almost devoid of all alloantibodies of their own origin. This is an important point to consider, especially when it becomes necessary to determine the blood groups of very young infants. Humans are born with an immature immunologic mechanism with respect to response to polysaccharide antigens that does not mature until approximately three months of age. Up to that time many alloantibodies present in their sera are of maternal origin, acquired through transplacental passage.

The naturally occurring anti-A and anti-B antibodies are most likely produced as a result of exposure to the normal environment. As pointed out previously, the A, B, and H antigens are ubiquitous in nature, being found in many strains of bacteria, animal dander, etc. The immunogenic stimulus afforded by these substances induces the production of cross-reactive antibodies of the type normally seen as naturally occurring antibodies.

The phenomenon of *immunologic tolerance*[7] is a mechanism that protects a person from responding to antigens found in his or her own body. Therefore, group A people who have A and H antigens produce only anti-B antibodies upon exposure to an A, B, and H laden environment. Individuals of group B make only anti-A upon the same exposure, and so on.

These antibodies are usually present in low titer with an optimal reaction temperature below 37C. Upon subsequent stimulation later in life, either through normal vaccination procedures that carry copious amounts of A and B-like antigens or through alloimmunization in pregnancy, people can form so-called immune anti-A and/or anti-B. These antibodies achieve high titers, are fully reactive at 37C, and may exhibit hemolytic properties. Thus when performing tests for anti-A and/or anti-B during routine blood-grouping determination, one must examine for the presence of hemolysis as well as agglutination.

The overall understanding of anti-A and anti-B is further complicated by the fact that the anti-A found in group B sera is of a different immunoglobulin class from that occurring in group O sera. In addition, the anti-A and anti-B found in the sera of people belonging to blood group O are accompanied by a third antibody called anti-A,B, which is present in fairly high concentration.

The anti-A,B is a cross-reactive antibody with a great deal of clinical importance since it has been implicated as the most likely causative agent in the ABO system of hemolytic disease of the newborn, a subject to be dealt with in the section on Rh. In addition, the anti-A,B found in group O serum is the antibody of choice for the detection of many of the weaker subgroups of A that fail to react with even the strongest example of anti-A. Because of this property, anti-A,B should be used along with anti-A and anti-B to determine the ABO blood groups in routine clinical practice.

LEWIS

The Lewis antigens, called Le^a and Le^b, are polysaccharide antigens that become adsorbed onto the surface of red cells. They are found principally in the saliva, serum, and other body fluids. The biochemical structure of these antigens, their relationships to the secretion of A, B, H, and the intimate relationship of the genetic pathway for their formation to the ABO system demand some mention of them at this point.

Intensive chemical studies have shown that the Le^a antigen is a glycoprotein with pyranose determinant groups. It is very similar in structure to the A, B, and H antigens, and thus may be synthesized in vivo from the same precursor substance. The genetic pathway for the production of the A, B, and H antigens of the erythrocyte has already been described. In all people, without regard to the secretor status, a certain amount of precursor is set aside for the manufacture of soluble glycoprotein antigens. Thus, all people have soluble antigens in their saliva and body fluids. Only the immunologic specificities of these antigens differ; secretors secrete A, B, or H and Le^b, nonsecretors secrete Le^a. To understand the inheritance of the Lewis antigens, the specific pathway dealing with the conversion of that portion of the precursor substance set aside for the manufacture of soluble antigens must be considered.

Four separate and genetically independent sets of alleles at four separate loci govern the production of the A, B, H, and Lewis antigens. The interaction of these four sets of alleles leads to the appearance of the appropriate antigens in the secretions. The Lewis antigens are then adsorbed onto the surface of the erythrocytes, depending on the quantity of each antigen in the plasma. The four sets of alleles taking part in this interaction are: 1. *A, B, O;* 2. *H, h;* 3. *Se, se;* and 4. *Le, le.* Each of the alleles codes for the production of specific glycosyl transferase enzymes that add a single sugar onto a glycoprotein backbone. The addition of each sugar results in the formation of a new serologic specificity. The genes *O, h, se,* and *le* are recessive amorphs, i.e., they do not control the synthesis of a particular enzyme and hence do not effect a change. The changes take place in a steplike fashion, and the order of reactivity based on present knowledge is: *Lele, Hh, Sese,* and *ABO.* Each alteration results not only in the production of a new antigenic specificity, but also in the formation of a new substrate on which the enzyme in the next step of the synthesis can act. The conversions that are effected by these enzymes do not exhaust the supply of substrate. Therefore, some of the by-products of a previous conversion are left behind. In addition, the presence of an amorph along the path can disrupt the synthesis, since the proper precursor will not be available for subsequent steps. Thus, the antigenic specificity depends on the action of the last gene in the sequence just before an amorph.

With the four sets of alleles, it is possible to construct twelve combinations of genotypes. These genotypes are shown in Table 13 along with the antigens that could appear both in the saliva and on the red cells of the individual. Apart from the hypothetic last two groups, representative examples of almost all of the phenotypes listed have been found. The phenotype frequencies of these antigens as detected on red cells are given in Table 14.

Immunochemical studies of the soluble antigens have resulted in the proposal of the tentative structures for the carbohydrate chains of these various blood group substances. These are shown in Figure 5. This diagram should make it evident that the Le^b antigen is an interaction product of the *H* and *Le* genes. It is also possible to see how both the H and Le^b specificities can be found in the secretions of the same individual. The glycosyl transferase responsible for applying the fucose onto the *n*-acetylglucosamine can do so only if *n*-acetylglucosamine is attached $\beta 1, 3$ to the terminal galactose. In the type 2 chain this linkage is not present. Therefore, the fucose is not attached, and the precursor is converted to the H determinant.

Nonsecretors who have at least one *Le* gene display Le^a antigen in their secretions regardless of the presence of the *H* gene. The *Se* genes are regulator genes that serve as *H* gene activators and the H genes in turn interact with the *Le* genes to form Le^b. Therefore, when an individual is *se/se* the *H* genes are either totally or partially

TABLE 13. GENOTYPES OF THE DIFFERENT KINDS OF SECRETORS

Secretor Status	Hypothetic Genotypes	Antigens on RBC				Antigens in Secretion			
		A or B	H	Le^a	Le^b	A or B	H	Le^a	Le^b
Normal secretor	A or B, H, Se, Le	+	+	−	+	+	+	+	+
	OO, H, Se, Le	−	+	−	+	−	+	+	+
Normal nonsecretor	A or B, H, sese, Le	+	+	+	−	−	−	+	−
	OO, H, sese, Le	−	+	+	−	−	−	+	−
Rare secretor	A or B, H, Se, lele	+	+	−	−	+	+	−	−
	OO, H, Se, lele	−	+	−	−	−	+	−	−
Rare nonsecretor	A or B, H, sese, lele	+	+	−	−	−	−	−	−
	OO, H, sese, lele	−	+	−	−	−	−	−	−
Bombay	A, B, or O, hh, Se or sese, Le	−	−	+	−	−	−	+	−
	A, B, or O, hh, Se or sese, lele	−	−	−	−	−	−	−	−

TABLE 14. PHENOTYPE FREQUENCIES OF LEWIS

Phenotype	White (%)	Black (%)
Le (a+b−)	22.00	23.11
Le (a−b+)	72.00	57.66
Le (a−b−)	6.00	19.22

inhibited, and the Le^a precursor is not converted to H substance. Since no H substance is formed there is no substrate available for the action of the enzymes that are controlled by the *A, B, O* genes. Thus, the only specificity detectable in the saliva of nonsecretors is Le^a.

Additional antigens of the Lewis system have been described, some of which are detectable on lymphocytes. These include Le^c and Le^d, as well as some that are expressed only in conjunction with certain ABO groups. They are beyond the scope of this discussion and the reader is referred to the recent work of Oriol.[8]

ANTIBODIES OF THE LEWIS BLOOD GROUP SYSTEM

Anti-Le^a and anti-Le^b are somewhat odd examples of blood group antibodies. They occur in the sera of most Le(a−b−) individuals as naturally occurring antibodies resulting from exposure to natural antigens. Some individuals of this phenotype produce an almost pure anti-Le^a and others an almost pure anti-Le^b. Still others produce antibodies that demonstrate cross-reactivity for both specificities.

Anti-Lewis antibodies, when mixed with the appropriate cell suspensions, behave as complete cold agglutinins, reacting well in saline solutions at an incubation temperature of 4C, and produce visible but extremely fragile clumps. On the other hand, saline suspensions of erythrocytes incubated at 37C are not normally clumped. Agglutination will occur with some examples of these agglutinins, however, if serum suspensions are used. Therefore, at 37C these antibodies can behave as typical incomplete agglutinins. When tests of this sort are carried out care must be taken in selecting the appropriate serum used for dilutions. For use with anti-Le^a the diluent must come from a person whose saliva or serum does not carry the Le^a antigen, otherwise neutralization of the antibodies will occur before they have a chance to react with the erythrocytes.

The antibodies of this system can bind complement. Thus, if fresh human serum of the appropriate type is added to an agglutination test as a source of complement, lysis will occur at 37C. With weak antisera the degree of lysis is markedly increased if the cells are trypsinized beforehand. The hemolytic activity is an important point. This characteristic, their high frequency, and their poor in vitro reactivity make these antibodies extremely dangerous from the standpoint of routine clinically applied blood transfusion, and hemolytic transfusion reactions have been reported.

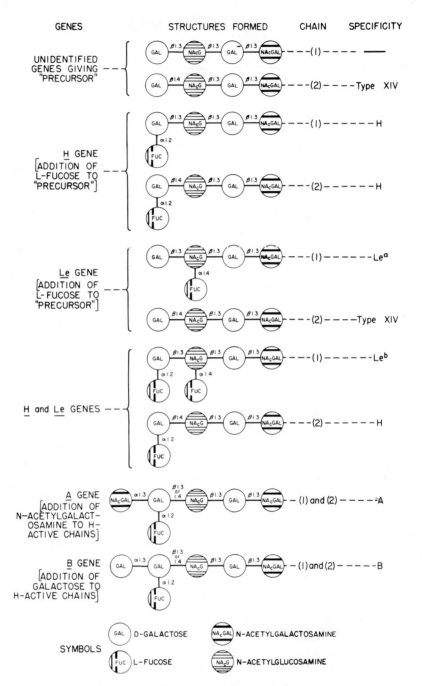

Fig. 5. The chemical structures of the A, B, H, and Lewis blood group substances resulting from sequential, gene-controlled fucosylation of the base chains. (*From Watkins. Science 152:178, 1966. Copyright 1966 by the American Association for the Advancement of Science.*)

The antiglobulin test as it is normally employed works poorly with these antibodies even when sera prepared against specific immunoglobulin classes are used. By far the best reactions are obtained if an anti-non-gamma antiglobulin test is employed with cells that have been exposed to antibodies in the presence of fresh serum as a source of complement. Because the Lewis antigens are not an integral part of the red cell membrane, it is possible to wash off the antigen-antibody complex during the antiglobulin procedure. However, it is known that complement is bound to the cell surface at a site adjacent to the antigen. This binding appears to be quite strong and, therefore, is not affected by washing steps. In such a manner it can serve as the antigenic receptor site for an anti-non-gamma Coombs serum.

In storage the antibodies are very unstable, and most people recommend that they be stored in the freeze-dried or lyophilized state. Instability of blood group antibodies is an unusual feature. One likely explanation for this peculiar characteristic is that these antibodies, unlike most other blood group antibodies, are made up of IgM immunoglobulin, which is known to be an unstable molecule capable of depolymerization in storage.

Rh BLOOD GROUPS

The second most important blood group system from the standpoint of clinical blood transfusion is the Rh system.

The Rh factor, described in 1940 by Landsteiner and Wiener,[9] was found as a result of injecting rabbits and later guinea pigs with the erythrocytes of the Rhesus monkey. Some of the resulting antisera reacted with the erythrocytes of approximately 85% of the random human population. This reaction was attributed to the presence of a new antigenic determinant shared by some humans and all Rhesus monkeys. Those cells that were agglutinated by the new antisera were termed Rh_o-*positive*, and those giving negative results were called Rh_o-*negative*.

A year earlier, Levine and Stetson[10] reported the recognition of an antibody in the serum of a mother who was delivered of a stillborn fetus. After delivery she suffered a severe transfusion reaction on receiving a unit of her husband's blood. They suggested that the mother had been immunized by an antigen inherited from the father and present on the red cells of the fetus but absent from her own erythrocytes. The antibody found by Levine and Stetson was shown to have the same specificity as the anti-Rhesus of Landsteiner and Wiener.

With the advent of increased blood transfusion in clinical medicine and more sophisticated serologic techniques, other antigens belonging to the Rh system were recognized by means of human alloantibodies, anti-C, anti-c, anti-E, and anti-e. Antithetic and genetic relationships were observed between the new and old antigens, so they were added to the system. Nevertheless, the original Rh antigen defined by human alloantisera, identical to that described by Levine and Stetson, which will be referred to here as D or Rh_o, is still the most important in the system. Individuals are separated into Rh_o-positive or -negative categories according to the reactivity of their cells with antisera having this primary Rh specificity.

After the antithetic relationship that existed between the antigens defined by the spectrum of antibodies in the Rh system was observed, two theories of inheritance were postulated. According to one theory, control of the system is achieved by three pairs of closely linked allelomorphic genes. These genes occupy three separate and distinct yet closely linked loci on each of a pair of chromosomes. Fisher and Race[11] called the genes, as well as the antigens they controlled, C and its allele c, E and its allele e, and D and its allele d. In this scheme the symbol D refers to the original and most important Rh antigen. Thus, anyone possessing the D antigen is said to be Rh_o-positive and anyone lacking it, Rh_o-negative. Despite numerous reports, no antiserum defining the product of the hypothetic d gene has been found. The term is used merely for the sake of convenience to express the absence of D. The genes at the three loci present on each one of a pair of chromosomes determine the expression of the corresponding antigens on the red cell surface.

Alternate alleles for the five major genes can be interjected into the system without changing the original genetic concept. According to Fisher the genes are arranged on the chromosome D-C-E. He suggested this after postulating genetic recombination as the explanation for the occurrence of the rare gene complexes CDE, CdE, and deletion as a cause of the phenotype –D–.

Another mode of inheritance set forth by Wiener[12] is the more generally accepted one, but the nomenclature is involved and unwieldy. To the neophyte who has access to only five standard anti-Rh sera (anti-D, anti-C, anti-E, anti-c, anti-e), the genotypic notation seems less explicit in relation to the antigens being defined by the reagents at hand and gives little useful information on the antigenic determinants present on a cell. Actually, the nomenclature is precise and makes some highly relevant distinctions between the chemical groupings that result from the action of certain genes and those determinants that finally combine with the antibodies. Wiener's theory of inheritance is based on the occurrence of multiple alleles at a single locus. In the terminology employed, the gene that occupies the locus is expressed on the red cell surface as an agglutinogen made up of an undefined number of antigenic determinants or factors, each of which can be detected with a specific antiserum. An example of this nomenclature is shown in Table 15.

Every agglutinogen or major antigen is a mosaic of many factors or determi-

TABLE 15. EQUIVALENT NOTIONS IN THE Rh BLOOD GROUP SYSTEM

Wiener		Fisher-Race	Shorthand Conversational
Agglutinogen	Factors		
Rh_o	**Rh_o, hr', hr''**	cDe	R^o
Rh_1	**Rh_o, rh', hr''**	CDe	R^1
Rh_2	**Rh_o, hr', rh''**	cDE	R^2
rh	**hr',hr''**	cde	r
rh'	**rh', hr''**	Cde	r'
rh''	**hr', rh''**	cdE	r''
Rh_z	**Rh_o, rh', rh''**	CDE	R^z
rh_y	**rh', rh''**	CdE	r^y

nants, not all of which need to be present for the substance to qualify as a particular agglutinogen.

If we consider only the five basic antigenic determinants distinguishable by the five standard Rh antisera, the two contrasting genetic theories of Fisher and Race and of Wiener can be illustrated diagrammatically with respect to chromosomal loci as shown in Figure 6.

One of the biggest problems in understanding and committing to memory the Rh-Hr nomenclature is that the symbols used try to convey the maximum amount of information. The letters R and h of the major symbol are supposed to denote that the antigenic determinants in question are without doubt a part of the Rhesus system. This leaves nothing more than the substitution of upper- and lower-case letters, superscripts, and subscripts to convey the most important message in the symbol.

A third nomenclature, free of genetic interpretation, has been suggested by Rosenfield et al.[13] This system uses numbers assigned to the antigens in the sequence of their discovery and permits the representation of the reactions of the cells with the antisera. Equal importance is given to both positive and negative results. A listing of the Rh antigens according to this scheme, along with a few representative examples, is given in Table 16. The phenotypes are expressed in terms of the reactions of the cells with each of the antisera preceded by the system symbol, which in this case is R followed by a colon. If a positive reaction is obtained with a particular antiserum, its number is listed in order. If a negative reaction is obtained, the number is listed preceded by a minus sign. If a weak reaction is obtained, the number listed is preceded by the letter w. If one is not fortunate enough to have access to all of the antisera, only the numbers of those reagents actually used are listed in numerical order.

As an example, the most common Rh phenotype among Caucasians may be given according to the three nomenclatures as follows:

Fisher-Race	CDe/ce
Wiener	R^1r
Rosenfield	R: 1, 2, −3, 4, 5

In the United States the CDE nomenclature is accepted as the standard primary nomenclature for clinical use.

DETERMINATION OF THE RH PHENOTYPES AND PRESUMPTIVE GENOTYPES

As previously stated, antisera capable of recognizing the five major antigens of the Rh system are the only ones routinely available to the usual clinical laboratory. The phenotype frequencies obtained with such sera are given in Table 17. On some occasions, however (to be elaborated on later), it becomes necessary to know whether the husband of an Rh_o-negative woman is either homozygous or heterozygous for

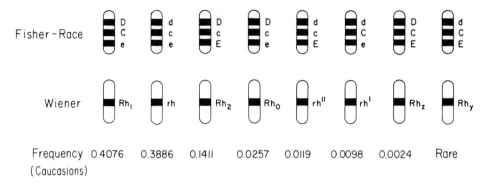

Fig. 6. Portions of the short arm of chromosome 1 showing the loci for Rh according to the theories of Fisher and Race and Wiener. The chromosomes are arranged from left to right in the descending order of their frequency in the population.

the allele conferring D (Rh_o). In the first case the capability of producing the D (Rh_o) antigen would be passed on to all of his offspring. In the heterozygous case, however, there would be a 50–50 chance of one half the offspring being Rh_o-negative (Fig. 7). The distinction between homozygotes and heterozygotes for alleles governing the production of the D (Rh_o) determinant cannot be made with absolute certainty in a given individual unless family studies are carried out, and sometimes not even then. However, a fairly accurate presumption can be made from the phenotypes as deduced from the reactions of the individual's red cells with the five standard anti-Rh sera and information on the relative frequencies of the various genotypes as deduced from family studies.

The following is the general procedure we have found useful for making the presumptive determination of the genotype (Table 18). The scheme is based on the relative frequencies of the eight basic chromosomal arrangements in the general population, which were listed previously in Figure 6. After the reactions of the cells with the antisera have been obtained, one tries to extract the most frequent combinations of antigens for the first chromosome; preference is always given to the chromosome carrying the *D* allele. The remaining antigens must be products of genes on the second chromosome, and only a *D* or *d* needs to be selected. The one selected should be the one that will complete the chromosomal arrangement that is most frequent.

ANTIGENIC MOSAICISM

Semiquantitative variation within the context of the D antigen can be observed. It will be noted that while the erythrocytes of certain individuals react with selected examples of anti-D, they do not react with all. In fact, there seems to be a definite range of reactivity extending from those that react weakly to those that absorb the antibodies but display visible reactions only after the antiglobulin test. Individuals whose cells behave in this fashion are called D^u.

TABLE 16. THE NUMERICAL Rh NOTATION AND ITS EQUIVALENTS[14]

Rosenfield	Fisher-Race	Wiener
Rh1	D	Rh_o
Rhw1	D^u	$Ⱦħ_o$
Rh2	C	rh′
Rh3	E	rh″
Rh4	c	hr′
Rh5	e	hr″
Rh6	f, ce	hr
Rh7	Ce and C^we	rh_i
Rh8	C^w	rh^{w1}
Rh9	C^x	Rh^x
Rh10	V, ce^s	hr^v
Rh11	E^w	Rh^{w2}
Rh12	G	rh^G
Rh13	no equivalent	Rh^A
Rh14	no equivalent	Rh^B
Rh15	no equivalent	Rh^C
Rh16	no equivalent	Rh^D
Rh17	no equivalent	Hr_o
Rh18	no equivalent	Hr
Rh19	no equivalent	hr^S
Rh20	VS, e^s	no equivalent
Rh21	C^G	no equivalent
Rh22	CE	no equivalent
Rh23	D^{wiel}	no equivalent
Rh24	E^T	no equivalent
Rh25	LW	no equivalent
Rh26	c^A (Deal)	Hr^A
Rh27	c^E	no equivalent
Rh28	Hernandez	hr^H
Rh29	Total Rh	RH
Rh30	Go^a, D^{Cor}	no equivalent
Rh31	no equivalent	hr^B
Rh32	Troll	R^N
Rh33	no equivalent	R_o Har
Rh34	Baas.	Hr^B
Rh35	1114	no equivalent
Rh36	Be^a	no equivalent
Rh37	Evans	no equivalent
Rh38	Duclos	no equivalent
Rh39	C-like	no equivalent
Rh40	Tar.	no equivalent
Rh41	Ce but not C^we	

The D^u classification is composed of two major types. The observed serologic reactivity of the two types is similar, but the reasons for the appearance of the antigen are apparently controlled by different underlying genetic mechanisms. A true D^u (*low-grade D^u*) is the direct product of an inherited gene. Therefore, a D^u characteristic of this type can be passed on to future generations. Ordinarily it can only be detected by the antiglobulin test after previously sensitizing the cells with anti-D sera. Individuals of this type can form anti-D on occasion.

**TABLE 17. PHENOTYPE FREQUENCIES
OF Rh**

Phenotype	White (%)	Black (%)
ccDEE	1.48	16.55
CCDEe	0.13	0.35
C^{w}CDEe	0.00	0.00
CCDee	18.17	2.82
C^{w}CDee	1.08	0.00
CCddEE	0.00	0.00
CCddEe	0.00	
C^{w}CddEe	0.00	0.00
CCddee	0.00	0.00
CdDEE	0.00	3.17
CcDEe	12.65	
C^{w}cDEe	0.27	0.00
CcDee	31.90	26.41
C^{w}cDee	0.54	0.35
CcddEE	0.00	0.00
CcddEe	0.00	
C^{w}cddEe	0.00	0.00
Ccddee	0.40	0.70
C^{w}cddee	0.00	0.00
ccDEe	12.11	
ccDee	2.42	43.31
ccddEE	0.00	0.35
ccddEe	0.27	
ccddee	18.57	5.99

　　　　The term *high-grade D^u* is used to identify cells that react weakly with either complete or incomplete anti-D and may on rare occasion require the use of the anti-globulin test for their demonstration. The apparent weakening of the D antigen in cells of such individuals is caused by a gene interaction phenomenon that is brought about by position effects. Thus, a gene controlling C in the trans position may suppress the D antigen on the opposite chromsome. Cells of the genotype *CDe/Cde* or *CDe/CdE* may give weak results with anti-D and appear as *CD^{u}e/Cde* or *CD^{u}e/CdE*. The high-grade D^u characteristic is not usually passed on to future generations, since only one chromosome is transmitted and the phenomenon depends on the infrequent *Cde* or *CdE* chromosomal arrangements. Individuals of this category do not form anti-D.

THE ANTIGEN G

The antigen G was recognized when a person was found whose cells reacted with sera containing anti-C along with anti-D (anti-CD) but not with pure anti-C or pure anti-D. The antigen characterized by these reactions was named G. Further

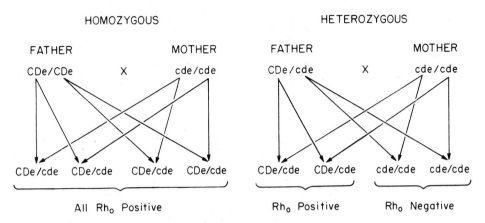

Fig. 7. Rh genotypes of children resulting from the mating of an Rh$_0$ negative mother with either a D-homozygous or D-heterozygous father.

investigation led to the discovery that cells possessing either the C or D antigen also had the G antigen. Later it could be shown that most anti-CD sera had an anti-G component and were really anti-C plus anti-D plus anti-G. In addition, many examples that appeared to be anti-CD were shown to be anti-D plus anti-G or, less commonly, anti-D plus anti-G. Further, it was demonstrated that the reaction of cells with anti-C or anti-D could be blocked by prior coating with anti-G.

This antigen, by itself, has little if any general clinical significance. However, it should be pointed out that many clinical laboratories use an anti-CD reagent for the diagnosis of the D antigen. The casual worker must be aware of the consequences of using such a reagent.

ANTIGENIC PRODUCTS OF ALTERNATE ALLELES

Many alleles and antigenic variants associated with *Cc* and *Ee* have been described. They are not of outstanding practical interest because of their infrequent occur-

TABLE 18. DETERMINATION OF THE Rh GENOTYPES

Cell Number	Reactions with with Antisera					First Chromo-some	Second Chromosome		Pre-sumptive Genotype
	D	C	E	c	e		1st Choice	2nd Choice	
1	+	+	−	+	+	CDe	cde	cDe	CDe/cde
2	+	−	+	+	+	cDE	cde	cDe	cDE/cde
3	+	+	+	+	+	CDe	cDE	cdE	CDe/cDE
4	+	+	−	−	+	CDe	CDe	Cde	CDe/CDe
5	+	−	+	+	−	cDE	cDE	cdE	cDE/cDE

rence but are of interest to many immunogeneticists. These alleles and variants were listed in Table 16. Further information is available in references 3, 14, and 15.

Rh DELETIONS AND Rh$_{NULL}$

Rare individuals have been found who lack one or all of the common Rh antigens. The genotype of such cells is written with a bar in the place of the missing determinant, for example: $cD-/cD-$, $C^W D-/C^W D-$, or $-D-/-D-$. Erythrocytes that lack antigenic determinants at the C and/or E locus, but possess the D antigen, have been shown to react much stronger with anti-D than do normal D-positive cells.

Originally it was felt that the phenotypes missing certain antigenic determinants represented a chromosomal deletion resulting from a split in the region between the loci for C and D and/or E and D. However, it has since been shown that such phenotypes may be the result of inhibitor or modifying genes.

Some extraordinary individuals have been reported whose red cells lacks all of the known Rh antigens. The term Rh$_{null}$ or—/— is applied to this cell type. The phenomenon can result from two different hereditary genetic effects: either the presence of recessive $X^o r$ genes that result in failure to produce substrate similar to h genes, or the presence of r genes that fail to convert a substrate such as the O genes.

The erythrocytes of Rh$_{null}$ individuals of both varieties suffer from a compensated hemolytic anemia. Levine has postulated that this is caused by a defect in the red cell membrane created by the absence of all Rh antigens. This idea is based on the assumption that the Rh antigens form an essential part of the membrane structure. Their absence, therefore, may create an architectural defect in the form of a perforation or a weakened spot in the membrane that results in premature erythrocyte destruction. Interestingly enough, the Bombay condition referred to in ABO does not result in anemia, probably because the ABH antigens are not an integral part of the membrane structure.

Rh ANTIBODIES

The recognition of Rh antibodies depends heavily on the serologic techniques available. The antibody of Levine and Stetson, which was the first recognized human example of anti-Rh, was a complete, 19S, IgM globulin antibody and, therefore, was capable of agglutinating cells suspended in saline. However anti-Rh antibodies are most commonly found as incomplete 7S, IgG agglutinins, so that the use of colloids as suspending media for serologic tests, the antiglobulin technique, enzyme methods, or other techniques designed to detect this form of antibody must be used for their demonstration.

The antibodies of the Rh system differ from those found in the ABO system in that they are products of definable alloimmunization rather than those circumstances provoking naturally occurring antibodies. Thus, as a general rule, Rh$_o$-negative individuals never have anti-Rh_0 antibodies, unless they have received an antigenic stimulus either through clinical transfusion, pregnancy, or some other means.

Rh GROUPS AND HEMOLYTIC DISEASE OF THE NEWBORN

Hemolytic disease of the newborn (HDN) is an acquired hemolytic anemia of the newborn characterized by a severe anemia with erythroid hyperplasia, splenomegaly, and hyperbilirubinemia. It has various clinical degrees, based on the severity of the symptoms. These range from a mild anemia with little or no visible jaundice to a disease of more severe proportions. Sometimes it can be severe enough to result in intrauterine death, with the subsequent delivery of a macerated fetus (hydrops fetalis). It has been shown that the greatest danger to the infant results from a deposition of bile pigments in the nuclei of the brain cells. This condition, known as *kernicterus* or, more recently, *bilirubin encephalopathy*, can result in permanent brain damage.

The firstborn child is rarely if ever affected. Sometimes the second child has a very mild case and the severity then increases with each subsequent childbirth, eventually leading to hydrops.

The pathogenic mechanism operative in this syndrome is an immunologic one, the direct result of alloimmunization of pregnancy. The mother, lacking some blood group antigen, usually D of the Rh system, is immunized by fetal cells that carry the D antigen inherited from the father. The resulting alloantibodies of the IgG class cross the placental barrier and react with the fetal erythrocytes, leading to their destruction (Fig. 8).

Alloimmunization of pregnancy and hemolytic disease of the newborn are not confined to the Rh blood group system. The potential for alloimmunization of a mother can exist whenever any blood group incompatibility exists, and thus antibodies may be produced to almost any of the red cell antigens or even the white cell antigens, as will be discussed later.

Not all blood group incompatible pregnancies result in HDN. It has been estimated that within the Rh system alone, alloimmunization with subsequent harmful sequelae occurs only 5% of the time that a suitable incompatibility exists. The lack of immunization is due to several factors, one of which is the relatively weak immunogenic ability of the antigens involved. Another is that the immune response is somewhat suppressed during pregnancy because of the secretion of various natural hormones.

The observation that there was a greater incidence of Rh antibodies in the sera of mothers who were of the same ABO group as their infants than in the sera of those women who were ABO incompatible has led to the development of a unique prophylactic treatment for Rh hemolytic disease. This finding could possibly arise from rapid removal of the fetus red cells from the maternal circulation by naturally occurring alloantibodies. It was reasoned that the primary and by far the largest immunizing stimulus comes from a massive transfusion of the mother with fetal blood during the trauma of parturition. Therefore, if a mother could be passively

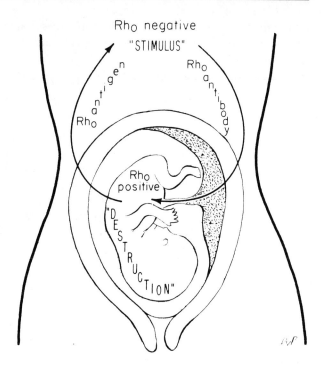

Fig. 8. Schematic representation of the pathogenic mechanism of hemolytic disease of the newborn. (*Adapted from Levine. Am J Obstet Gynecol 42:925, 1941.*)

immunized with Rh antibodies during a period shortly after delivery, the anti-Rh antibodies would act like anti-A or anti-B and help remove the fetal cells before they could exert an antigenic stimulus. Accordingly, Rh immune globulin prepared from high-titered anti-Rh sera is now administered prophylactically to all Rh_o-negative women who give birth to Rh_o-positive infants and who have no demonstrable antibodies. Since this practice was initiated there is a significantly lower incidence of anti-Rh antibodies in Rh_o-negative women at the time of their second pregnancy and the procedure is considered successful.

Although the mechanism by which this protection operates is still obscure, it is known that the procedure protects against primary immunization but is ineffectual against a secondary response. The use of this substance has been extended to protect against immunization after transfusion of Rh_o-positive blood into an Rh_o-negative recipient. However, substantially larger doses must be given because of the relatively larger quantities of incompatible red cells involved.

OTHER BLOOD GROUP SYSTEMS

In addition to the clinically important ABO system and the related Lewis and the Rh systems, there are a large number of other red cell alloantigens and systems.

Some of them can have clinical significance when patients form antibodies as a result of transfusion or pregnancy. Others have significance only in forensic or genetic applications. They will be mentioned here, but for a detailed discussion of each, the reader is referred to related works.[3, 15]

MNSs Antigens

The MNSs is a system of two very closely linked loci, M and S, each with two major alleles, *M, N* and *S, s,* along with a large number of variants (Table 19). The genotypic makeup of an individual is readily discernible from the phenotypes in a family study.

TABLE 19. PHENOTYPE FREQUENCIES OF MN

Phenotype	White (%)	Black (%)
M	29.22	25.25
N	21.1	27.00
MN	49.66	47.74
S	11	3
Ss	44	28
ss	45	69

For the most part, M and N are detected with sera produced in animals by deliberate immunization and purification by absorption. The M and N antigenic specificities are determined by the presence of carbohydrate antigenic structures and therefore can be detected with certain lectins. *Vicea graminea* can be used to detect N and *Iberis amara* is specific for M. Antibodies to S and s can be found as alloantibodies produced as a result of transfusion or pregnancy.

Occasionally people are found whose cells fail to react with either anti-S or anti-s. They are called U negative. They can produce an antibody, anti-U, which reacts with the cells of any person possessing either S or s. Since most people fall into this category, they present a problem in selecting compatible blood for transfusion. At present there is a nationwide registry of U negative individuals who can serve as suitable donors.

P Antigens

The P blood group system (Table 20) is composed of three major alleles, P_1, P_2, and *p*, which give rise to the genotypes P_1P_1, P_1P_2, P_1p, P_2P_2, P_2p, and *pp*. Only *pp* individuals are truly P negative and they constitute only a small percentage of the population. Weak antibodies to P_1 may be formed as a result of exposure to cross-reactive antigens present in the environment. These antibodies, in addition to being weak, react preferentially in the cold.

Immune antibodies to antigens of the P system, especially those with the combined specificity anti-P, $P_1 + P^k$, can fix complement and pose serious clinical problems.

TABLE 20. PHENOTYPES, POSSIBLE GENOTYPES, AND APPROXIMATE FREQUENCIES OF P_1, P_2, AND p

Phenotype	Possible Genotypes	Approximate Frequency (%)
P_1	$P_1 P_1$	30.0
	$P_1 P_2$	50.0
	$P_1 p$	> 0.1
P_2	$P_2 P_2$	19.0
	$P_2 p$	> 0.1
p	pp	> 0.1

Kell Antigens

Originally only two antigens were ascribed to the Kell blood group system, K (Kell) and k (Cellano) (Table 21). Both of these antigens are capable of provoking a brisk immune response in transfused patients and pregnant women who lack the responsible antigens. The antigen Kell occurs in only 9% of all individuals in either the homozygous (genotype KK) or the heterozygous (genotype Kk) condition, leaving 91% of the population susceptible to alloimmunization by this antigen. Since only one in 500 persons lacks the k (Cellano) antigen, the production of anti-k is much less frequent but becomes clinically more urgent in those rare instances when it is necessary to obtain k-negative (KK) blood to transfuse a patient who has been immunized by this antigen.

The K and k antigens are exceptionally good immunogens. Consequently, formation of anti-K antibodies as a result of transfusion or pregnancy occurs with some degree of regularity. It is only because of the relative frequencies of the antigens in the population that anti-K and anti-k do not cause clinical difficulties more frequently and are not considered significant in the routine clinical sense.

Since its original description, several other antigens have been found associated with this system. They are Kp^a (Penney), Kp^b (Routenberg), and Js^a and Js^b (Sutter).

Anti-K and anti-k can cause severe, even fatal, hemolytic transfusion reactions and hemolytic disease of the newborn.

The anti-K antibody is normally an incomplete antibody that fails to agglutinate red cells suspended in saline. The most reliable method for demonstrating anti-K or anti-k reactivity is the indirect antiglobulin test, although some examples of anti-K can best be detected with anti-gamma globulin Coombs sera. Others,

TABLE 21. PHENOTYPE FREQUENCIES OF KELL

Phenotype	White (%)	Black (%)
K	0.24	Rare
Kk	6.65	2.0
k	93.10	98.0

TABLE 22. DUFFY GENOTYPES AND PHENOTYPES

Genotype	Phenotype	Reaction with Antisera		Frequency	
		Anti-Fy^a	Anti-Fy^b	White (%)	Black (%)
$Fy^a Fy^a$	Fy (a+b−)	+	−	19.58	8.8
$Fy^a Fy^b$	Fy (a+b+)	+	+	47.86	1.6
$Fy^b Fy^b$	Fy (a−b+)	−	+	32.56	21.6
Fy Fy	Fy (a−b−)	−	−	0.00	68.0

mainly composed of IgM, are best detected with anti-non-gamma reagents. Anti-K has been shown to be capable of binding complement; therefore, occasional hemolysis may be seen in vitro in the presence of fresh serum. This property makes the antibody extremely dangerous in vivo, since it can cause rapid intravascular hemolysis.

Duffy Antigens

The genotypes and phenotypes of the Duffy blood groups are given in Table 22. A high percentage of blacks fail to react with either anti-Fy^a or anti-Fy^b, thus appearing to belong to a phenotype Fy(a−b−). It is believed that these individuals are homozygous for a third allele in the system called *Fy*, which produces an antigen designated Fy^4.

An interesting facet of Duffy is that blacks who are Fy(a−b−) have a natural resistance to malaria. The work of Miller et al.[16] indicates that red cells carrying the Duffy antigen produced by this phenotype cannot be invaded by the malarial parasite *Plasmodium vivax*. This implies that such erythrocytes lack a particular receptor that is required for the attachment and subsequent penetration by the parasite.

For the most part, anti-Fy^a antibodies are found in the sera of multitransfused patients, formed as a result of specific stimulation. The typical anti-Fy^a antibody is a warm-reacting incomplete agglutinin that requires the use of the antiglobulin test for its demonstration.

Anti-Fy^b is one of the most poorly documented antibodies, so it is difficult to assess its clinical significance other than to speculate that as an immune antibody it would be capable of causing both hemolytic disease of the newborn and transfusion reactions.

Kidd Antigens

The two antigens of the Kidd system whose genotypes and phenotypes are shown in Table 23 were thought for many years to be inherited in a simple codominant manner. The genetics are complicated since people have been described who are Jk (a−b−). As an explanation for this phenotype, it can be assumed that there exists either a third silent allele, Jk (the product of which is undetectable), or a modifying

TABLE 23. KIDD GENOTYPES AND PHENOTYPES

Genotype	Phenotype	Frequency White (%)	Black (%)
Jk^aJk^a	Jk (a+b−)	24.47	57.0
Jk^aJk^b	Jk (a+b+)	52.68	34.0
Jk^bJk^b	Jk (a−b+)	22.85	9.0
Jk Jk	Jk (a−b−)	Rare	—

gene that exerts a suppressive influence on the antigenic expression of Jk^a and Jk^b. These Jk (a−b−) individuals have been found exclusively among Asians and their descendants; however, there is evidence that a silent Jk gene may also be present in the Caucasian population.

Anti-Jk^a is not an uncommon antibody formed as a result of transfusion or pregnancy. It is often found in a serum in conjunction with antibodies of other specificities. Many, although not all, examples of anti-Jk^a are complement-dependent. Therefore, a serum suspected of containing anti-Jk^a should be tested while active complement is present. Fresh normal serum may be added to a stored serum as a source of complement, but this may dilute a weak antibody and result in a false negative reaction. The use of ficin- or trypsin-treated cells will generally result in enhanced reactions with anti-Jk^a, especially if the indirect antiglobulin test using a broad spectrum reagent to detect the non-gamma proteins is employed as well.

Most examples of anti-Jk^a react best by the indirect antiglobulin technique. Anti-Jk^b, like anti-Jk^a, is usually found in conjunction with antibodies belonging to other blood group systems and is best detected by the use of the antiglobulin test.

Both anti-Jk^a and anti-Jk^b can cause severe transfusion reactions. The titer of these antibodies tends to fall rapidly in vivo, making it undetectable in routine compatibility tests. Because of this unusual production of anti-Jk^a, during transfusion therapy a preimmunized patient may experience a brisk anamnestic response to small amounts of antigenic stimulus. The results of this response are manifested by a severe delayed transfusion reaction that may occur hours or days after the blood has been administered. This proves that a negative compatibility test is not an absolute guarantee of freedom from adverse reactions.

The Lutheran Antigens

The major significance of the Lutheran blood group system is that the genetic locus controlling expression of its antigens is linked to the ABH secretor locus. As such, Lutheran-secretor is the first example of autosomal linkage in humans. The system is composed of two primary alleles, Lu^a and Lu^b, which give rise to the phenotypes shown in Table 24.

The phenotype Lu(a−b−), discovered in 1961, defies adequate explanation thus far. The usual explanation, the existence of a third allele, Lu, is unsatisfactory since no quantitative evidence for the existence of an Lu gene has been found. Tentatively, the existence of a low frequency but dominant suppressor gene, called

TABLE 24. PHENOTYPE FREQUENCIES OF LUTHERAN

Phenotype	White (%)	Black (%)
Lu (a+)	0.01	
Lu (a+b+)	7.9	4.86
Lu (b+)	99.94	

In(Lu), has been postulated. This is not the only answer, however, since some families carry an Lu(a−b−) phenotype that can be attributed to a recessive characteristic.

Therefore, there are two null phenotypes in this system. One of these is the result of dominant genes while the other is caused by recessive genes.

A large number of Lutheran-related "para-Lutheran" antigens has been described, largely as a result of the zeal native to most blood group workers. The supposed alleles have been assigned numbers ranging from Lu^4 to Lu^{20}. Aside from Lu^1, which is Lu^a, Lu^2, which is Lu^b, and Lu^3, which corresponds to Lu^{ab}, and the alleles Lu^6 and Lu^9, the question of whether or not the remainder are true antigens controlled by alleles associated with the Lutheran system is not fully answered.

Not very many examples of anti-Lu^a antibodies have been found and it is a matter of speculation as to whether they are all products of active immunization, since they react best at room temperature with saline cell suspensions.

On the other hand, numerous examples of anti-Lu^b have been reported that are serologically quite different from anti-Lu^a. For the most part they are incomplete agglutinins that react best at 37C by the antiglobulin technique. An interesting finding has been that several examples of anti-Lu^b are IgA immunoglobulin.

I Antigens

The I antigen is found on the red cells of practically all normal adults. The nonspecific cold agglutination found in the sera of patients as a result of certain types of viral infections or in patients suffering from cold antibody type acquired hemolytic anemia reacts with this antigen. The antigen seems to be a maturation antigen since newborn infants do not possess it. They have another antigen called i. Thus the antigen I differs from other blood group antigens because of its slow maturation, its almost universal occurrence, and the qualitative difference between positives and negatives (Fig. 9).

This system has no clinical significance in blood transfusion. However, it frequently causes problems in the blood bank laboratory and workers must be cognizant of its existence.

Other Erythrocyte Antigens

Apart from the systems described in this section there are several other systems as well as an entire array of alloantigenic markers of red blood cells (Table 25). Some

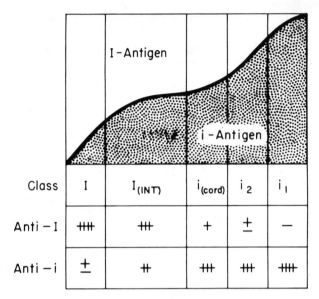

Class	I	I$_{(INT)}$	i$_{(cord)}$	i$_2$	i$_1$
Anti − I	+++	+++	+	±	−
Anti − i	±	++	+++	+++	+++

Fig. 9. Theoretical amounts of I and i antigen in the different classes of I-positive cells.

of the other systems, such as Diego, are important only as anthropologic tools. The antigen Xg^a, on the other hand, is an important genetic marker since it is transmitted via alleles situated on the X sex chromsome rather than on one of the autosomes. Therefore, it can be used as a reference point for mapping the X chromosome. A number of antigens apart from P and I are found in the vast majority of the human population. These are the Public Blood Group Antigens, an example of which is the antigen Vel. Similarly there are others that are restricted to a certain population or even to a family, such as Kamhüber. The reader is referred to related works for a more complete discussion of this subject.[3, 15]

The T antigen is universally present on the red blood cells of all individuals, but the antibody-combining site is buried by other chemical structures. However, when the erythrocytes are subjected to the action of bacterial proteolytic enzymes these determinants are uncovered and can combine with antibodies. As it turns out, the sera of all individuals contain an anti-T. Therefore, it is obvious that anyone who has an overwhelming bacterial septicemia, with massive doses of enzymes in his or her circulation, will have red cells that can react with all reagent antisera, all normal sera, and indeed even with his or her own serum.

It is currently popular to refer to erythrocytes that have acquired this property as polyagglutinable red cells, which describes any situation in which the affected cells are agglutinated by most but not necessarily all normal sera even if the responsible antigen-antibody system is known.

Apart from the T antigen a number of other antigens have been implicated, including Tk, which may be a transition phase in either the development or repression of T; Tn, which seems to be an acquired red cell membrane defect that is permanent and may involve other hematopoietic cells as well; and Cad, which in reality may be a very common blood group surface antigen (Sd^a) to which a large proportion of the normal population may have antibodies under the appropriate conditions.

TABLE 25. PUBLIC BLOOD GROUP ANTIGENS

h	Ola Ware	Mz 443
Vel	Holly (Hy)	Sisson
Gerbich (Ge)	Dp	Snyder
Lan-So^a	August (At^a)	Gonsowski (Gn^a)
H$_T$	York (Yk^a)	En^a
Yussef (Yus)	Cipriano	Knops-Helgeson (Kn^a)
Stirling (Cs^a)	Bradford	Jr^a
Chido	Gallner	Ge:1
Gregory (Gy^a)	Henry	Jo^a
El	Kelly	

PRIVATE BLOOD GROUP ANTIGENS

Levay	Traversu (Tr^a)	Torkildsen (To^a)
Jobbins (Job)	Webb (Wb)	Skjelbred
Becker	Kamhüber-Far	Peters (Pt^a)
Ven	Jn^a	Moen (Mo^a)
Berrens (Be^a)	Radin (Rd)	Wade
Romunde (Rm)	Gladding	Zd
Batty (By^a)	Hunt (Ht^a)	Reid (Re^a)
Chr^a	Donaviesky	Jensen (Je^a)
Swann (Sw^a)	E. Amos	Ahonen (An^a)
Stobo	Terrano	Hov
Biles (Bi)	Thoms (Th^a)	Hey
Box (Bx^a)	Heibel	Roselund (Rl^a)

LESS WELL-DOCUMENTED ANTIGENS

Bp^a	Cross	Orriss
Ls	McAulay	Sullivan
Yahuda	Br 726750	"Evans"
Finlay	Rich	Fleming
Black	Gon	Per
Car	Griffiths	Savior
Tod	Hollister	Wetz
Vennera	Marriott	Kosis
Winbourne	Peacock-Mansfield	Mar
Wil	Ken	

Review Questions

1. The greatest amount of H antigen is found on red cells of which blood group?
2. If the Mother is A CcDe and the Father is O Ccde, what are the possible blood groups of the baby?
3. Give the equivalent of the following in the Wiener terminology: *CdE, cDe, CDe, cDE, cde.*
4. What set of antibodies would you anticipate finding in a patient with no history of transfusion or pregnancy?

5. From what is Anti-A$_1$ Lectin obtained?
6. What is the explanation if an Rh$_o$-positive father and an Rh$_o$-negative mother have an Rh$_o$-negative child?
7. What is the D^u factor?
8. Why are prenatal antibody titers useful?
9. What is a person said to be if like genes are inherited from each parent?
10. Give the Fisher-Race equivalents of the following: **rh**″, **hr**′, R^1, R^o, R^z.
11. What is the most likely antibody specificity if a patient is found to be group A$_1$ with an antibody that agglutinates A$_2$ cells but not A$_1$ cells?
12. When do we say that a person is homozygous for the **rh**′ factor?
13. List two causes of the D^u factor.
14. What can be concluded from the appearance of an Rh antibody in the serum of an Rh$_o$-negative woman during her second pregnancy?
15. What designates an individual as Group A?
16. When are most blood group antigens developed?
17. Explain the Hardy-Weinberg equilibrium.
18. What is the significance of the binomial distribution with respect to genetic events?
19. Describe the difference between a genotype and a phenotype.
20. How is genetic information translated into blood group antigenic structures?

REFERENCES

1. Morton NE: Sequential tests for the detection of linkage. Am J Hum Genet 7:277, 1955.
2. Hackel E: The Emily Cooley Lecture: Population Genetics and Human Blood Groups. In A Seminar on Basic Genetics. Houston, Texas, AABB, 1969.
3. Race RR and Sanger R: Blood Groups in Man. 6th ed. London, Blackwell, 1975.
4. Bhende YM, Despande CK, and Bhatia HM et al: A "new" blood-group character related to the ABO system. Lancet 1:903, 1952.
5. Ceppellini R: Physiological genetics of human blood group factors. In Wolstenstrolme GEW, O'Conner CM (eds): Symposium on the Biochemistry of Human Genetics. London, Churchill, 1959.
6. Watkins WM and Morgan WTJ: Possible genetical pathways for the biosynthesis of blood group mucopolysaccharides. Vox Sang 4:97, 1959.
7. Roitt J: Essential Immunology. 4th ed. London, Blackwell, 1980.
8. Oriol R, Danilovs J, Lemieux R, Terasaki P, and Bernoco D: Lympho-cytotoxic definition of combined ABH and Lewis antigens and their transfer from sera to lymphocytes. Hum Immunol 1:195, 1980.
9. Landsteiner K and Wiener AS: An agglutinable factor in human blood recognized by immune sera for Rhesus blood. Proc Soc Exp Biol Med 43:223, 1940.
10. Levine P and Stetson RE: An unusual case of intragroup agglutination. JAMA 113:126, 1939.
11. Fisher RA and Race RR: Rh frequencies in Britain. Nature 157:48, 1946.
12. Wiener AS, Gaven JA, and Gordon EB: Blood group factors in anthropoid apes and monkeys. II. Further studies on the Rh-Hr factors. Am J Phys Anthrop 11:39, 1953.

13. Rosenfield RE, Allen FH Jr, Swisher SN, and Kochwa S: A review of Rh serology and presentation of a new terminology. Transfusion 2:287, 1962.

14. Issitt PD: Serology and Genetics of the Rhesus Blood Groups System. Cincinnati, Montgomery Scientific Publications, 1979.

15. Zmijewski CM: Immunohematology. 3rd ed. New York, Appleton-Century-Crofts, 1978.

16. Miller LH, Mason SJ, Clyde DF, and McGinniss MH: The resistance factor of plasmodium vivax in blacks. The Duffy-blood-group genotype, Fy Fy. N Engl J Med 295:302, 1976.

CHAPTER 6

Diagnostic Tests

Objectives

By reading this chapter the student should learn the:
1. Basic principles of donor-recipient matching for blood transfusion.
2. Consequences of a transfusion of incompatible whole blood.
3. Importance of the ABO and Rh blood groups in transfusion.
4. Purpose of and methods used in antibody screening.
5. Rationale underlying the cross-match procedure.
6. Methods used in resolving incompatible cross-matches.
7. Significance of good clerical methods and the positive establishment of identity.
8. Specific causes of the three major types of transfusion reactions.
9. Methods used in the diagnosis of hemolytic disease of the newborn and its prophylaxis.

DONOR BLOOD SELECTION FOR TRANSFUSION

The basic principles employed in donor selection for transfusion today were originally described in 1911.[1] The most deleterious incompatibility, often referred to as the major incompatibility, is one in which antibodies are present in the recipient's plasma that are reactive with the donor's red cells. This can be understood readily by considering the events that take place during the transfusion of blood (Fig. 1).

From a mechanical point of view, a transfusion is administered intravenously and the donor blood is allowed to gradually drip into the venous circulation of the recipient. As a result, exceedingly small quantities of antigen-bearing red cells are constantly being added to the large pool of antibodies contained in the entire circulating volume of the recipient. These conditions allow ample opportunity for antigen to meet antibody, resulting in rapid and constant antigen-antibody interaction with a concomitant destruction of red cells. By the time the transfusion has been completed a total volume of approximately 200 ml of donor red cells will have been destroyed.

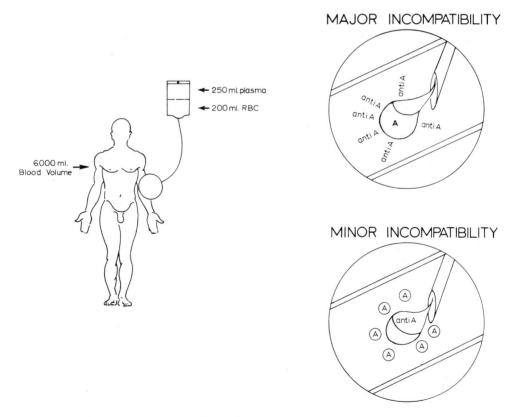

Fig. 1. This cartoon graphically depicts the logic underlying the principles of blood donor selection and transfusion. For explanation see text.

A large quantity of free hemoglobulin is released from this volume of red cells, which of itself is neophrotoxic and contributes to renal failure. Associated with this is the fact that a massive antigen-antibody reaction with associated complement activation has occurred. This results in the formation and release of a host of vasoactive substances that alter capillary blood flow, seriously compromise the circulatory system, and initiate a series of events that lead to shock.

These physiologic events cause the symptoms of a hemolytic transfusion reaction, i.e., severe hemoglobinuria ("urine as black as soot")[2] followed by total anuria, pain in the lower back, elevated temperature, uricaria, dyspnea, a feeling of impending doom, and, if untreated, shock and eventual death.

When incompatible transfusions are given some of the clinical symptoms become apparent when as little as 55 cc of whole blood is given. However, if the recipient is under general anesthesia, the symptoms are almost totally masked. This makes transfusions given during extensive surgery especially dangerous. Unfortunately most transfusions need to be administered under such conditions since surgery cannot be performed without blood loss and required replacement. Therefore, appropriate donor selection and matching in the laboratory are of critical importance.

Without question, the ABO blood groups of donor and recipient are the primary consideration in any transfusion of whole blood. This should be eminently clear from the fact that all people, without exception, carry antibodies in their plasma with a specificity reciprocal to that of the antigens on their erythrocytes.

In contrast to the overwhelming importance of the major compatibility, the antithesis, or minor incompatibility, i.e., antibodies in the serum of the donor reactive with antigens on the red cells of the recipient, is of little or no consequence. Under these conditions, small amounts of antibodies contained in the donor plasma being infused drop-by-drop encounter an excessively large antigen excess represented by the recipient's total red cell mass. Because these conditions do not favor efficient binding of antibody to antigen, very little such binding takes place. After the transfusion is complete, the antibody concentration in the donor plasma is reduced through dilution by the recipient's blood volume. This dilution can approximate 1:24, considering that the 250 ml of plasma containing antibodies in one unit of blood is incorporated in the 6,000 ml blood volume of an average-size adult patient.

In the specific case of the ABO blood groups, a dilution of 1:24 is beyond the effective titer of the naturally occurring anti-A and/or anti-B antibodies present in a normal donor. In addition, absorption of the antibodies to antigens found in the vascular endothelium of the recipient and neutralization by soluble blood group substances found in the plasma of recipients who are secretors diminish the effectiveness of the transfused antibodies even further.

In normal practice, consideration of the minor incompatibility can be totally avoided by transfusing only within the ABO groups: group O blood is given only to group O recipients, group A blood to A's, etc. Under certain unusual circumstances, however, it may not be possible to adhere strictly to these rules. In such cases it is permissible to make use of the principles just described.

Since the major incompatibility to be avoided is one in which the recipient has

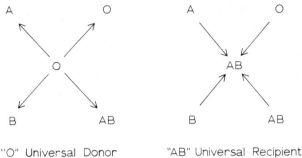

    "O" Universal Donor   "AB" Universal Recipient

Fig. 2. A useful scheme to illustrate the principles of transfusions as they apply to the universal donor and the universal recipient. Since no one can form antibodies to the group O antigen, the red cells of this group can be given to any of the four groups. Group AB individuals do not possess antibodies against any of the other groups and therefore can receive blood of any of the four groups.

antibodies reactive with antigens on his or her red cells, it can be concluded that group O blood can be safely transfused to any member of the four groups. This is possible because group O cells do not contain either the A or the B antigens and therefore neither anti-A nor anti-B can react with them. The group O donor thus has been termed the *universal donor*. In the same context, the individual who belongs to group AB, since he or she has neither anti-A nor anti-B, can receive blood of any of the other groups and may be considered a *universal recipient* (Fig. 2).

It must be stressed that these circumstances pertain only to situations involving the ABO blood groups. And even in these cases exceptions do occur that preclude the use of these rules without reservation. For example, as pointed out earlier, the level of naturally occurring anti-A and anti-B frequently increases as a result of immunization with bacterial vaccines. In today's world, it is difficult to find people with low levels of isoagglutinins because of the widespread use of prophylactic vaccination. Group O blood administered without due concern for the level of antibodies in its plasma can create conditions amenable to the destruction of the recipient's own red cells.[3] Although this does not always result in a fatal hemolytic reaction, it is counterproductive to the therapeutic regimen. For this reason, universal donor blood is most frequently administered as packed red cells from which all of the plasma containing antibodies have been removed. This gives the recipient the advantage of the antigen-free red cell mass without the potential dangers of antibodies.[4]

In life-threatening emergencies, however, whole blood of group O that previously has been ascertained to contain relatively safe levels of anti-A and anti-B (<1:100) may be administered with extreme care.

Because of the low frequency of group AB in the general population, it often is difficult to find an ABO identical donor. In the cases it is acceptable to use the concept of the universal recipient. To keep the possibility of a minor transfusion reaction to a minimum, blood of either group A or group B is selected for transfusion. It is generally accepted that anti-A is more dangerous than anti-B. Therefore, group AB recipients are generally transfused with group A rather than group B blood.

In the normal course of standard operating procedures, further donor selection is performed to preclude immunization that might compromise the patient for one reason or another. The D (Rh_o) antigen of the Rh blood group system is probably the second most powerful immunogen among the various blood group antigens. Apart from causing problems with subsequent transfusions, immunization of women of child-bearing age to this antigen can cause severe problems in subsequent pregnancies should the resultant fetus be D (Rh_o) positive. Therefore, consideration of D (Rh_o) is given in donor selection for transfusion.

As a rule, D (Rh_o) negative recipients are given only D (Rh_o) negative blood. On the other hand, D (Rh_o) positive recipients can safely receive either D (Rh_o) positive or D (Rh_o) negative blood. However, because D (Rh_o) negatives are less frequent in the population and therefore less frequent among donors, D (Rh_o) negative blood is generally reserved for O D (Rh_o) negative recipients.

Special consideration must be given to people who, rather than being simple D (Rh_o) positives, are the variant class of D^u. As mentioned previously, these people fall into two categories, the gene interaction type who are genetically D but whose red cell expression of this antigen is suppressed, and those who are genetically D^u. Although both of these classes of individuals behave differently with respect to their ability to induce antibody production in D (Rh_o) negative individuals and their ability to respond themselves to D antigen, no distinction is made in the classes in clinical transfusion. In other words, all individuals whose D antigens are detectable only by means of the indirect antiglobulin test are considered D^u.

In the past it was required that all individuals (both recipients and donors) be tested for the presence of the D^u variant whenever they appeared to be D negative in routine testing. Now it is sufficient to test only donors. Therefore, according to current acceptable standards D^u recipients are regarded as D (Rh_o) negative and receive D (Rh_o) negative blood,[4] since certain D^u individuals can develop anti-D antibodies of restricted specificity if they are challenged with D antigen.

On the other hand, donors who are D (Rh_o) negative must be tested for the presence of D^u. If D^u is shown to be present irrespective of its origin, the donor is considered D (Rh_o) positive and his or her blood given only to D (Rh_o) positive recipients, since the D^u antigen of either the genetic or gene interaction type can induce the formation of anti-D antibodies in D (Rh_o) negative individuals.

No attempt is made in current practice to protect against immunization by any of the other Rh antigens, such as C, c, E, or e. Experience has shown that the frequency of this event is so low as to be of no serious consequence except in very specialized cases.

These procedures apply to the appropriate selection of donors within the ABO and Rh blood group systems. It should be eminently clear, however, that humans have a vast number of alloantigens apart from these groups. A complete consideration of each of these alloantigens in donor selection would preclude the possibility of ever being able to transfuse.

Two conditions prevail that allow routine transfusion to be performed. First, with few exceptions, naturally occurring antibodies reactive with red cell antigens at body temperature do not occur outside of the ABO blood group system. Patients who have never been exposed to blood group immunization by transfusion or pregnancy theoretically should not present a major incompatibility problem. Second, for the most part the majority of antigens belonging to the other blood group systems are relatively weak immunogens. Immunization with subsequent antibody formation does not usually occur under the conditions of a normal blood transfusion. Usually the patient is debilitated from the illness requiring the transfusion in the first place, so the immune system is not functioning at optimal capacity. In addition, blood is frequently administered to patients who are actively bleeding, so the offending antigens do not have the opportunity to exert an immunologic stimulus during the period of time that may be required to achieve an immune response. Finally, the intravenous route is not a very satisfactory route of immunization. In spite of these factors, however, immunization can occur occasionally, especially if a particular recipient requires extensive transfusion therapy over an extended period of time. Therefore periodic antibody screening of such patients is recommended to detect such an occurrence.

ANTIBODY SCREENING

A person receiving a blood transfusion can have a hemolytic transfusion reaction only if antibodies reactive with red cell antigens and the red cells bearing those antigens are present in his or her circulation simultaneously. Furthermore, the two components, antibodies and red cells bearing antigens, must be present in the appropriate concentrations to allow an antigen-antibody reaction to take place.

Not all intravascular red cell antigen-antibody reactions lead to rapid intravascular hemolysis. For this to occur complement must be activated by the reaction, which does not appear to be a property universal among blood group antibodies. Therefore, this type of reaction is primarily associated with the complement-binding antibodies of the ABO, Lewis, Kell, Kidd, and sometimes P blood group systems.

Antibodies produced to other blood group antigens, such as those of the Rh system, are not very efficient complement activators. As a matter of fact, some of the antibodies produced as a result of stimulation with these antigens belong to the IgG_2 or IgG_4 subclasses, which interact with complement poorly or not at all. Red cells coated with antibodies of this class are physiologically removed by the spleen. Although this results in a less violent reaction than that experienced with intravascular hemolysis, it is no less severe in its consequences.

According to how donors are selected for transfusion apart from ABO and Rh and the polymorphism of blood group antigens, there is bound to be some antigenic incompatibility between the recipient and the donor, i.e., the donor red cells are almost certain (by pure chance alone) to carry antigens that are lacking in the donor. Therefore, some form of antibody response must be expected from every transfu-

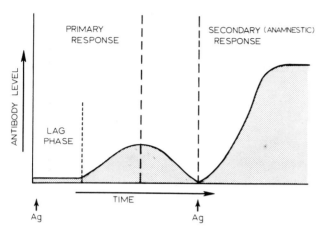

PRIMARY RESPONSE

SECONDARY (ANAMNESTIC) RESPONSE

LAG PHASE

ANTIBODY LEVEL

TIME

Ag

Ag

Fig. 3. A profile of the typical antibody response to immunization with blood group antigens. After a lag phase, during which the immune system is triggered into action, antibodies of primarily the IgM class gradually begin to appear, reach some level, and then begin to fall off. A second dose of antigens results in a very brisk appearance of antibodies that are mostly IgG. The final antibody level attained is considerably higher and may persist for long periods of time.

sion. This should not be taken to imply that such a response will occur in every case, but that it should be expected.

A primary antibody response to antigens administered in a given unit of blood is of little or no consequence during the course of that particular transfusion. According to the dynamics of the primary response, there is a delay of from five to ten days before antibodies first begin to appear (Fig. 3). When they finally do appear they are present in low concentration and so may be effectively diluted by the recipient's circulation. Usually by the time the antibody concentration has reached a significant level, the transfused red cells, which have a half life of approximately twenty-seven days, are almost completely gone from the circulation.

Even though a primary antibody response causes little if any difficulty with the transfusion that results in its induction, it is important to be aware that the event has occurred and to note it in a patient's transfusion record. The reason for this is that such individuals, on a second exposure to even a very small number of red cells from a subsequent transfusion, can mount a brisk secondary or anamnestic response. When a secondary response occurs, a high concentration of antibodies may develop within a very short period of time, which may be as brief as twenty-four hours. Under these circumstances an ample volume of transfused red cells may be present, especially if the patient is not actively bleeding. This can lead to what is often termed a delayed transfusion reaction.[5]

Delayed reactions are particularly dangerous because they are totally unexpected. For example, a patient could apparently tolerate the transfusion well, exhibiting no adverse symptoms. Then quite suddenly and sometimes at a time when he or she is completely unattended, the patient experiences the symptoms of a transfusion reaction.

These events can be avoided in part by adopting the principle that a thorough and a priori knowledge of the antibodies to all blood group antigens present in a recipient's serum is essential to safe transfusion and a logical basis for donor selection. This can be achieved by antibody screening, i.e., testing the serum of potential recipients for the presence of all varieties of blood group antibodies.

Previously it was stated that for the most part antibodies present in the plasma of the donor directed against the recipient's red cell antigens were practically innocuous. Several reasons were given for this: the antibodies were frequently present in low concentrations and therefore were effectively diluted; the antibodies were preferentially neutralized by soluble antigens in the plasma of secretors, rendering them ineffective against red cells; and finally, they could be absorbed by antigens present on the surface of other cells such as those of the vascular endothelium. At the same time it was pointed out that these factors were true if the antibody concentration in the donor plasma was low enough. It also must be pointed out that this reasoning holds true only for antibodies within the ABO blood group system.

Antibodies to other blood group antigens produced as a result of pregnancy or transfusion are frequently of a higher titer than that which is considered safe; their respective antigens are confined to the red cell membrane so tissue absorption cannot take place and soluble antigens do not occur. Therefore, even though such donor antibodies rarely produce classical hemolytic transfusion reactions, they can combine with recipient red cells and cause an increased rate of destruction. This defeats the main purpose of the blood transfusion and must be avoided.[6]

Apart from the decreased survival of the recipient's own red cells due to donor antibodies, certain other hazardous conditions can occur when multiple transfusions are given. It is entirely possible for a donor to have antibodies that fail to react with the recipient's red cells because of a lack of the appropriate antigen. On the other hand, the red cells of the donor of a second transfusion may contain the appropriate antigen. Therefore, when the second transfusion is given, the recipient may experience a reaction caused by the effects of the passively infused antibodies from the first transfusion combining and causing the destruction of the red cells of the second transfusion. This is called the *incubator effect,* since the recipient's own immune status has nothing to do with the reaction, and he or she merely acts as the vessel in which the reaction occurs.[7]

Problems associated with unexpected antibodies occurring in potential transfusion recipients as well as those associated with antibodies in donor plasma can be avoided by means of thorough screening of the sera of both recipients and donors for the presence of antibodies to blood group antigens other than those of the ABO system. Such antibodies are frequently referred to as *irregular antibodies,* although the term *unexpected antibodies* is more precise.

Donor plasmas are normally screened for the presence of unexpected antibodies at the time of each donation. Patient sera are usually screened before the first transfusion is administered and, if continual transfusions are to be given, at suitable intervals, usually every forty-eight hours, to detect the appearance of antibodies that may have arisen as a result of the transfusions given previously.

Regardless of whether the serum is of donor or recipient origin, the antibody screening is performed in the same way. First, the serum is tested with two different suspensions of group O erythrocytes that carry representative examples of all the antigens against which most blood group antibodies found in clinical practice are formed. The cells selected should be as heterozygous as possible so that most of the gene products of the established blood group systems are represented between them. In addition, if it is possible, appropriate cells should be selected for screening that carry representative examples of all of the public specificities as well as some of the private ones.

The serologic techniques selected for this type of antibody screening should be the most sensitive available, but more importantly, they should be capable of detecting all clinically relevant forms of antibody. All workers in the field of serology are constantly in search of the most sensitive techniques. For example, shortly after the discovery of the antiglobulin test, many investigators felt that it was the most sensitive serologic method, and, therefore, its use could ensure the detectability of all incomplete antibodies. However, sensitivity is only relative and is highly dependent on the particular antigen-antibody system under study. A technique that is very sensitive in one system may be very insensitive or even ineffective in another. This behavior is influenced by a number of factors other than the immunoglobulin class of the prevalent antibody. For example, even though IgG antibodies directed against the Rh antigens appear to be incomplete agglutinins, in blood group systems other than Rh, the distribution of serologic activity according to immunoglobulin class is not clear. This is especially true of the ABO system, in which there are many examples of anti-A and anti-B, especially those found in the sera of group O individuals, that are 7S, IgG, but behave as complete agglutinins, causing clumping of the appropriate erythrocytes in saline suspending media. Similarly it is possible to find examples of immune anti-A that may also be 7S, IgG, but that are incomplete, requiring the presence of normal adult human serum to produce visible cell clumping.

In some instances, even antibodies composed of IgM immunoglobulins, such as those of the Kidd and Lewis systems, may on occasion behave as incomplete agglutinins. Therefore, it should be clearly understood that the immunoglobulin class is not the only determinant of serologic reactivity. Other factors, such as the location of the particular antigenic receptor site and its chemical configuration, as well as other yet unknown physical conditions, must undoubtedly play an important role in determining the degree of sensitivity of a particular serologic test for the optimum detection of antibodies to a given blood group system. To encompass the potential antibody spectrum, saline tests for complete antibodies as well as Low Ionic Strength Solutions LISS and antiglobulin tests for incomplete antibodies are generally carried out.

Donor or recipient sera that fail to react with either of the two cells under the stringent conditions employed are considered to be devoid of clinically significant antibodies. On the other hand, sera that react by any of the techniques with either one or both of the screening cells contain such an antibody. Should this be the case, under ordinary circumstances it is beneficial to determine the specificity of the antibody or antibodies involved.

If the antibody is found in a donor's plasma, the plasma containing it should be removed and the unit administered as packed cells. The identification of the antibody specificities in such material can result in a potentially useful source of typing serum.

Information pertaining to the specificity of the antibodies in a recipient's serum is necessary to make an intelligent decision about proper donor selection. For example, it may be found that the antibody is anti-k. Therefore, k (Cellano) negative blood will be required for transfusion. Since the frequency of this type is only one in 100 the likelihood of having an appropriate unit in the blood bank inventory may be small. The clinician treating the patient can be informed that a delay in obtaining a suitable donor is inevitable, thereby allowing appropriate steps to be taken in postponing therapy or surgery. In the meantime, knowing the specific type of donor blood required makes it easier to obtain it from other sources.

Antibody identification in its simplest form consists of testing the serum containing the antibody against a test cell panel, which is a selected collection of red cells from about ten or twelve different donors. Such panels of red cells are readily available from commercial sources but can be prepared in any laboratory that has access to a large number of completely typed volunteers.

The red cell donors for this type of panel are selected in such a way that each of the well-recognized blood group antigens is represented in several of the cells and simultaneously there are a number of cells that completely lack the antigen. A typical cell panel is illustrated in Table 1. In this example the D antigen is found on five of the cells and absent from the remaining six cells. The C antigen is present on four cells and absent from six cells, etc.

Since antibodies to the various antigens of the Rh system are the ones most frequently encountered either singly or in combination with antibodies to some of the remaining blood group antigens, their occurrence could mask the presence of another antibody. Therefore, the combinations of antigens represented by the individual cells must be carefully selected.

The serologic tests used in this procedure are as critical to the appropriate identification of antibodies as is the make-up of the test cell panel. All modern systems used to establish the antibody specificity of an unknown serum call for subjecting it to a battery of techniques under different environmental conditions (saline, LISS, antiglobulin, enzymes, @ 4C, 22C, and 37C). These recommendations are based on sound principles of serologic detective work and on observations that have been made over a long period of time.

The discovery of additional blood group systems, coupled with an ever-increasing number of tests designed for the detection of incomplete antibodies, has resulted in a "rule of thumb" classification of blood group antibodies based on their particular mode of reactivity under laboratory conditions. It has been observed that saline agglutinins reactive at 22C are most likely anti-A or anti-B, anti-M or anti-N, or anti-P if the reaction is strongest at 4C. Antibodies reacting in high-protein diluents or LISS are most often associated with the Rh system while those demonstrable only by the antiglobulin technique usually are anti-Kell or anti-Duffy. Although this rule of thumb is useful, the points presented on the sensitivity of serologic reactions should not be forgotten.

After the serum is tested with the cells and each of the reactions noted, the overall reaction pattern (distribution of positives and negatives) of the serum with all of the cells in each of the serologic techniques employed is compared with the pattern of presence or absence of each of the antigens in all of the cells. In this manner a first attempt at identification can be made. Table 2 depicts the reactions

TABLE 1. THE DISTRIBUTION OF ANTIGENS IN A TYPICAL PANEL COMPOSED OF ELEVEN SELECT CELLS FOR ANTIBODY IDENTIFICATION

Cell Donor	D	C	E	c	e	Cw	M	N	S	s	K	k	Kpa	Jsa	P1	Lea	Leb	Fya	Fyb	Jka	Jkb	Lua
1. 461	0	0	0	+	+	0	0	+	+	+	+	0	0	0	+	+	0	+	0	0	+	0
2. 318	0	0	0	+	+	0	+	+	+	0	0	+	+	0	+	0	+	+	0	+	+	0
3. 291	0	0	0	+	+	0	+	+	0	+	0	+	0	0	0	0	0	0	+	0	+	0
4. 479	0	0	0	+	+	0	+	+	+	+	0	+	0	0	0	0	+	+	+	+	0	0
5. 138	0	+	0	+	+	0	+	0	+	+	0	+	0	0	+	+	0	0	+	+	0	0
6. 666	0	0	+	+	+	0	0	+	0	+	0	+	0	0	+	0	+	+	0	+	+	0
7. 340	+	+	0	0	+	0	+	+	0	+	0	+	0	0	0	0	0	0	0	+	+	0
8. 285	+	+	0	0	+	+	+	+	0	+	+	+	0	+	0	0	+	+	0	0	+	+
9. 316	+	+	0	0	+	0	0	+	0	+	0	+	0	0	+w	0	+	0	+	+	+	0
10. 521	+	0	+	+	0	0	0	+	+	0	+	+	0	0	0	0	+	+	+	0	+	0
11. 212	+	+	0	+	0	0	+	0	+	0	0	+	0	0	+	+	+	+	0	+	+	0

Note: Cell 6 is Di(a+). All cells are positive for Kp^b, Js^b, and Lu^b.

TABLE 2. REACTIONS OF AN UNKNOWN SERUM CONTAINING ANTI-D WITH THE CELL PANEL

Cell Donor	D	Reactions of Unknown Serum	Interpretation
1	0	0	
2	0	0	
3	0	0	
4	0	0	
5	0	0	
6	0	0	
7	+	+	
8	+	+	anti-D
9	+	+	
10	+	+	
11	+	+	

of a serum containing an unknown antibody with the eleven cells of the panel. It can be seen that the reactive pattern of the unknown corresponds exactly to the distribution of the D (Rh$_o$) antigen among the cells of the panel. Therefore, it can be concluded that the unknown antibody is anti-D.

This type of direct comparison works well if the serum contains an antibody for only one blood group specificity. Frequently, however, the sera of patients, especially those who have been heavily transfused, contain more than one antibody. Even in such cases, though, it may be possible to discern the identities of both antibodies if the antigen patterns of the cells are appropriate. If this is not possible, a well-constructed panel may provide data that will allow an educated guess to be made as to the true identities of the antibodies involved. A careful inspection of the reactions of the unknown serum shown in Table 3 reveals that some of the positives could be explained by the presence of anti-D (below the line). When the reactions with the D-positive cells are subtracted, a pattern emerges that matches that of the

TABLE 3. REACTIONS OF AN UNKNOWN SERUM CONTAINING TWO ANTIBODIES WITH THE CELL PANEL

Cell Donor	D	Fy^a	Reactions of Unknown Serum	Interpretation
1	0	+	+	
2	0	+	+	
3	0	0	0	anti-Fy^a
4	0	+	+	
5	0	0	0	
6	0	+	+	
7	+	0	+	
8	+	+	+	anti-D
9	+	0	+	
10	+	0	+	
11	+	+	+	

occurrence of the Duffy (Fy^a) antigen around the remaining cells. Therefore it can be concluded that in all probability the serum contains two antibodies, one of them anti-D and the other anti-Fy^a. When this occurs additional cells must be selected for a second panel in which the distribution of antigens will allow each of the antibodies to be distinguished more precisely. In the example just given, a special panel consisting of several D-positive, Fy^a-negative cells, D-negative, Fy^a-negative cells, and D-negative, Fy^a-positive cells would be required.

If this fails, more sophisticated methods such as absorption and elution must be performed. These procedures are normally carried out in reference laboratories and require a considerable amount of time, expertise, and appropriate reagents.

Under ordinary circumstances, unless the reactions of the serum containing the antibody are straightforward, the identification obtained as the result of screening alone should be considered preliminary. Such a preliminary identification is adequate for clinical use, since in the case of a patient, a final cross-match will be performed, and in the case of a donor, the blood ordinarily will be administered as packed cells. On the other hand, if the serum containing the antibody is to be used as a source of reagent for future blood-grouping tests or perhaps for investigational purposes of one kind or another, further confirmatory tests are obligatory.

One of the problems associated with the test cell panels routinely employed is the lack of an adequate number of cells representing the antigens of lower frequency. Clinical panels are designed to offer the highest discriminating power with the smallest number of cells for the sake of efficiency. Therefore, even though they may contain five cells that are positive for D and five that are negative for the antigen, they may have only one cell positive for Js^a. A serum that reacts only with the Js(a+) cell may be a true example of anti-Js^a. On the other hand, it is possible that this single reaction was caused either by some technical error or by a heretofore unknown antigen that happened to be on the Js(a+) cell as well. Therefore, a confirmatory test would be done on a panel specifically designed to identify Js^a. Such a panel might consist of five Js(a+) cells and five Js(a−) cells. Obviously, confirmatory tests in such cases are beyond the scope of routine clinical laboratories since they require access to a vast array of suitable test cells.

CROSS-MATCH PROCEDURES

The foregoing discussion can be summarized by saying that suitable blood for transfusion is selected according to the ABO and Rh groups of the recipient. Further precautions are taken to preclude any dangerous consequences resulting from donor antibodies against either the recipient or another donor's red cells by adequate antibody screening and plasma removal if necessary. Finally, antibody screening on the recipient's serum is performed to uncover the existence of and identify any unexpected antibodies that might have been formed as the result of some unknown immunization.

Despite these precautionary steps, the possibility still remains that some type of incompatibility might exist between the serum of the patient and the red cells of the donor selected for transfusion. To determine with a reasonable degree of certainty that this is not the case it is customary to perform a specific compatibility test or cross-match with every donor prior to transfusion.

The cross-match test itself is nothing more than a serologic test performed between the serum of the recipient and the red cells in the particular unit of blood to be used. Obviously the most sensitive methods capable of detecting clinically significant antibodies must be employed. When this test is performed properly even the slightest degree of agglutination or hemolysis is an indication that an in vivo transfusion reaction could occur and thus the specific donor blood should not be used.

There are a number of reasons for such a reaction to occur, the most obvious being that: a. the red cells of the donor carry an antigen that was not represented in the screening panels and to which the recipient has an antibody; b. the most recent serum sample of the recipient used for the cross-match has antibodies that reached detectable levels since the last antibody screening was performed; or c. perhaps there is a clerical error associated with the transcription of the ABO blood group of the recipient or the intended donor. In any case, the particular unit of blood cannot be used for the transfusion of the patient in question and another unit must be selected and appropriately cross-matched.

The occurrence of an incompatible cross-match test invariably results in a state of anxiety in the blood bank laboratory. The clinicians, anxious to help their bleeding patients, are eagerly awaiting the receipt of blood for transfusion. The technologist begins to feel guilty and doubtful about the results of the test. Finally, since other patients are waiting to get their cross-matches performed, a backlog occurs in the workflow while the current problem is considered. Within the framework of this chaos the blood bank technologist must retain a modicum of logic, order, and self control.

The first step to be taken in all instances of cross-match incompatibility is to ascertain that the serum sample on hand and used for the cross-match belongs to the patient in question. If there is even the slightest doubt, a new sample must be obtained without delay. Second, as many additional units of blood belonging to the appropriate ABO and Rh group as possible should be selected and all of the cross-matches repeated. Nine times out of ten these cross-matches will result in the discovery of some units of blood that are nonreactive and can be safely administered. Then, when the patient's blood needs are satisfied and the atmosphere of the laboratory returns to a state of relative tranquility, the question of why the original cross-match was incompatible can be addressed and resolved.

As a general policy all incompatible cross-matches should be appropriately resolved and the solution properly noted in the patient laboratory record for future references, so the problem can be avoided altogether when the same patient requires additional blood.

The test between the serum of the recipient and the red cells of the donor is known as the *major cross-match,* and will detect those antibodies that can result in a rapid destruction of donor cells leading to a hemolytic transfusion reaction. Before the advent of routine donor antibody screening, some laboratories performed *minor cross-matches,* i.e., tests of the donor serum versus the recipient's red cells. However, adequate donor antibody screening and plasma removal from positive units eliminate the need to perform this additional test. Furthermore, the test is meaningless when the principles of either the universal donor or the universl recipient are used, since the donor sera in these cases would contain either anti-A, anti-B, or both and the minor cross-match would be positive.

For the cross-match to adequately predict the safe outcome of a particular transfusion, it is imperative that the serum sample of the recipient adequately reflects his or her antibody status at the time the transfusion is to be given. For this reason, blood samples of the patient (pilot tubes) to be used for cross-match purposes should be collected as close to the time of the intended transfusion as possible. In most cases this should be no earlier than forty-eight hours before the transfusion is to be given. This does not mean, however, that the blood group determinations and antibody screening cannot be performed well in advance. As a matter of fact, such practice is to be encouraged to allow enough time for these tests to be performed and interpreted at a leisurely pace and still allow enough time to resolve any difficulties well before the transfusion is actually required. Generally speaking, it is difficult to set hard and fast rules for a specific timetable since timing can vary somewhat depending on the circumstances. Therefore, the blood bank director must be consulted to establish a policy and set the appropriate guidelines.

There is one instance, however, when definite guidelines can be established— the person who is receiving chronic blood transfusions. These patients usually receive one or two units of blood daily for several successive days or over an extended period. Such circumstances can occur in the case of patients suffering from aplastic anemia who require constant transfusions, or sometimes in major surgical cases that require prolonged periods of recuperation. Patients in either of these categories might require ten or more transfusions during a typical hospital stay. Obviously in cases such as these the serum sample collected for testing before the first transfusion does not adequately represent the antibody content of the patient's serum after four or five units of blood have already been given.

This is true for a number of reasons. First, under the conditions just described at least a third or more of the patient's own plasma would have been replaced by plasma from a number of different donors. Any single one of these might have contained some kind of previously undetected antibody against infrequent antigens that were absent from the panel but might be found on the red cells of the subsequent donors and form the basis of a reaction. Second, any of the first several units could have initiated a primary immune response resulting in the production of new antibodies that could then react with donor red cells given later on in the course of transfusion. Although this would be an unusual circumstance, certainly many courses of chronic transfusion last long enough for a primary response to occur. Finally, one of the transfusions could cause an anamnestic antibody response so that undetectable levels of antibodies might be increased quite abruptly to dangerous levels. These could cause severe reactions if the transfusions were continued in sequence without pausing to repeat the cross-matches with fresh patient serum samples collected at suitable intervals.

The cross-match is considered by many as the single most important pretrans-fusions serologic test, since it allows a direct observation of the consequences of mixing the patient's sera with the red cells to be transfused. As a result most insti-tutions and the AABB standards clearly stipulate that a transfusion cannot be given without appropriate cross-matching except in life-threatening emergencies as spe-cifically attested to by a physician. Even in these cases a retrospective cross-match must be performed as quickly as practicable.[4]

CLERICAL METHODS AND ESTABLISHING IDENTITY

Contrary to expectation, the majority of transfusion reactions that occur in a mod-ern hospital are not caused by technical or laboratory problems—they are the di-rect result of clerical errors.

Clerical errors can be numerous as well as insidious in any large hospital be-cause of the number of people and services associated with a given patient's case. The similarity in the names of different people and the frequent inability of the pa-tient to communicate properly either because of illness or ignorance of the proce-dures that are being performed invite clerical errors. Consider for a moment the sit-uation that occurs daily in the clinical chemistry laboratory. More than 800 tubes of blood of 300 patients arrive first thing in the morning. These are codified in some way, separated into tubes containing serum and cells, and dispatched to the various sections for testing. The results of the measurements then have to be incorporated with the proper names and locations and the results returned to the patients' charts.

Even under the most stringent controls occasional mix-ups do occur. As far as the majority of lab tests are concerned, these mix-ups may result in delay or some minor inconvenience to the physician or to the patient. However, this is not true in the blood bank, where even a minor mix-up could result in a fatal reaction. There-fore special precautions are taken with blood bank samples from phlebotomy to in-fusion to preserve the identity of the patient and the donor. Extreme care must be exercised to ensure that the regulations instituted to safeguard the patients' welfare are not violated in any way and exceptions should not be tolerated.

Most of the established rules for identification may vary from institution to in-stitution, but they are all designed to secure three major points. First, that the donor blood sample used for laboratory testing is exactly the same as that in the container to be used for transfusion, and that this blood is that which circulated in the veins of the donor himself or herself. Second, the patient's blood sample is ex-actly the same blood as that circulating in the veins of the patient himself or herself. Finally, the unit of blood that was tested with a particular recipient's blood sample in the laboratory is given to no one else except the intended recipient.

It is evident that a variety of systems can be devised, but, in general, the simpler the system the better. Further, regardless of how complex or how simple the system may be, its success depends solely on the acccurate recording of identifiers and the subsequent reading and checking of these identifiers at every step of the whole transfusion process. In the usual course of business it is often tempting to assume certain things, e.g., that a tube of blood placed in a rack and momentarily left unattended is still the same one found there upon returning. Such an attitude can be ill afforded, since in that interval the tube or even the entire rack for that matter could have been interchanged with another by a fellow worker. Therefore the identification on the tube must be rechecked prior to its use and nothing can be assumed.

Identification of Donors

Donors are normally identified in the bleeding facility by a unique alphanumeric code. This number appears on all records pertinent to the donor, e.g., donor history, address, time of last donation, association with a donor club, etc. Modern collection methods make use of plastic blood bags that have an integral donor tube through which the blood is collected. These donor tubes have an indelibly imprinted container number placed repeatedly on their surface by the manufacturer. After the blood is collected, this donor tube is pinched off and sealed at intervals, creating a series of segments each carrying the container number. Segments prepared in this fashion are then used as the pilot samples of donor blood for cross-matching and blood grouping. This insures that the blood being tested is the same as that which is in the bag and eventually will be given to the patient.

The blood-collecting facility keeps a record of the container number into which a given donor was bled, making it possible to trace the blood in a segment to the container itself and then to the donor. In the operation of the transfusion service, the primary consideration is that the blood for testing comes from the specific unit that will be transfused, and strict attention to segment members is mandatory.

Patient Identification

Patients in a modern hospital are normally identified by an admission number as well as their name, each of which is placed on an identifying bracelet. Before a pilot sample is collected from a patient it is essential to check the bracelet not only for the name but also for the number. If the patient is coherent, it is considered good practice to ask his or her name. In large institutions especially, several patients may have similar or even identical names. In addition, it is common to move patients from one bed to another in semiprivate rooms, so that locations are a poor indicator of identity.

To ensure the continuity of identification, it is good practice for the person who collects the blood sample to sign the label on the tube along with a witness who has verified the identification. In this way positive identification is maintained throughout all testing procedures.

Finally, when the cross-matched unit of blood is delivered to the patient's bedside, donor and patient identification must be rechecked. Again, the person starting the infusion should attest to the fact that such an identity check was performed, and should enter this along with the date and time at which the transfusion was started into the permanent patient record.

THE PROBLEM CROSS-MATCH

Occasionally patients are encountered whose sera react with the red cells of every donor tested. The strength of this reactivity may vary from very weak and discernible only by microscopic examination to quite strong. This situation creates a serious problem, since these patients often are seriously ill and usually require frequent transfusion. Since a nonreactive cross-match is a prerequisite to a transfusion, how can the laboratory ascertain that no in vivo reaction will occur in the face of such blanket reactivity? There are a number of steps that can be taken to ensure the patient's safety based on the cause of this abnormal serologic behavior, which may be due to any of several underlying factors.

The previous discussion should make it obvious that one of the most logical explanations could be that the patient's serum contains true antibodies to blood group antigens. The serum could either contain antibodies of a single specificity directed against a high frequency antigen that is expected to occur in the majority of the populations, such as Vel or U, or it could contain a variety of antibodies with different specificities directed against a number of different antigens and therefore mimic an antibody to a public blood group specificity. In either of these two cases the problem is readily solved once the identity of the antibodies in the serum has been established through antibody screening or referral to a reference service for more sophisticated testing. If the serum does contain a monospecific antibody to a high frequency antigen such as Vel or U, donors negative for these antigens can be acquired by contacting a national registry of rare donors. If, on the other hand, the serum contains a multispecific mixture of antibodies, the selection of donors negative for each of the offending antigens should solve the problem.

On a more practical level it must be remembered that the patient's serum containing antibodies is the richest source of typing reagent and it itself can be used to "type" donors. Therefore, if enough donors are available, they can be cross-matched, and frequently a compatible one can be located unless the offending antigen is directed against one of the true public specificities.

Apart from those instances when a positive cross-match is caused by specific antibodies to a high frequency antigen or to a number of different antigens, there may be a whole series of cases in which no antibodies displaying blood group specificity can be implicated. This group of cases can be roughly classified according to the serologic phase or specific circumstances in which the cross-match is positive. The reaction may be said to be caused by cold agglutinins, warm agglutinins, and/or autoagglutinins.

Patient sera containing cold agglutinins are frequently encountered in the blood bank laboratory. A large proportion of the normal population has low levels of anti-I antibodies that react at only slightly reduced temperatures. In addition, the antibodies are made in response to infection with organisms that sometimes are associated with the common cold, which is prevalent during the winter. Finally, some patients may actually be suffering from an autoimmune hemolytic anemia of the cold antibody type.

Antibodies of this variety become most troublesome during two seasons of the year, midwinter and midsummer, and are caused primarily by laboratory conditions and only secondarily by the patients themselves. One of the frequently employed serologic phases of the cross-match procedure includes some form of incubation at room temperature. During the offending seasons, the room temperature of most hospital laboratories is below normal; in the winter because of inadequate heating and in the summer because of excessive air conditioning. This decrease in room temperature is just enough to cause cold agglutinins to become active.

The majority of cold agglutinins, even those with anti-I specificity, can be easily identified. These antibodies will readily agglutinate adult red blood cells at refrigerator temperatures. However, when they are incubated at 37C, the agglutination disappears, only to recur upon cooling. These antibodies are hardly ever of clinical significance since the recipient of the transfusion is normally at 37C, a temperature that is not conducive to binding by these antibodies. Occasionally certain steps are taken to warm the blood before infusion. Such precautions are usually unnecessary if the recipient's body temperature is normal. When they are taken, however, they must be done by approved methods to avoid damaging the blood. Patients who have cold agglutinins should not be transfused under conditions of hypothermia.

Two special cases of cold antibodies that can give the impression of being nonspecific are worthy of note—the situations encountered when either anti-A_1 or anti-H are involved. Anti-A_1 occurs in the sera of some individuals belonging to group A_2 and A_2B while anti-H may occasionally be found in the sera of some group A_1 and A_1B individuals. Both of these antibodies react at low temperatures and on occasion can give the impression of nonspecificity due to the existing circumstances. For example, most of the group A donors in the normal blood bank are group A_1. Therefore the serum of a group A_2 patient who has an anti-A_1 will react with most if not all group A donors. By the same token most group A_1 cells and all group A_2 cells will react with anti-H to some degree. Therefore a "super" A_1 patient's serum containing anti-H will likewise react with all group A donors in the bank. Because anti-A_1 and anti-H, which behave like cold agglutinins in vitro, can on occasion be hemolytic in vivo, it is unwise to ignore them. Therefore, the sera of group A patients who display "nonspecific" cold agglutinins should be suspect.

Patients' sera that react in vitro with all donor red cells at 37C are referred to as having panagglutinins. They may react broadly due to a number of causes, including specific and nonspecific factors ranging from blood group antibodies as well as other immunoproteins to nonantibody agglutinating factors produced by the patient as a direct result of the disease or of the therapeutic modality being employed. They may include the anti-T antibodies, described elsewhere, that react with red cell determinants exposed by the in vivo or in vitro enzymatic activity of bacterial organisms; antibodies to caprylate preservatives in the albumin preparations used for serologic tests; antibodies to penicillin that will agglutinate red cells coated with this antibiotic; abnormal proteins produced as a result of therapy with such drugs as Aldomet or Apresoline, which are known to coat red cells and give a false positive direct antiglobulin test; paraproteins produced as a result of multiple myeloma and other malignancies that alter the viscosity of the serum and act on the second stage of agglutination; or autoantibodies in the warm antibody type of autoimmune hemolytic anemia.

Although each of these represents a problem of great magnitude that can be diagnosed correctly only by an experienced reference laboratory, the problem cross-match itself can be resolved from a practical standpoint by a number of approaches. One of these is to attempt to absorb out the nonspecific panagglutinin. This is a practice that can lead to difficulties since the major problem associated with panagglutination is that it may mask a specific antigen-antibody reaction. Although absorption can remove the unwanted panagglutinin, the danger of removing the specific antibody as well remains a potential threat in such a procedure.

Another approach is to use the patient's own red cells in a control cross-match along with the usual combination of patient's serum and donor's cells. Theoretically, at least, if the patient's serum contains a nonspecific panagglutinin along with a specific antidonor antibody, the degree of agglutination observed with the specific donor should be greater than that obtained in the control. Therefore, if the reaction observed with the donor is no greater than that observed with the patient's own cells, the donor is probably compatible. This procedure is based on logic and it does not always guarantee an uncomplicated transfusion. However, in certain cases it is the best that can be done.

The ideal solution to the problem in such cases is to perform a clinical cross-match. First, using the patient control method, the very best donor (i.e., the one whose red cells are agglutinated the least) is selected. Then a small sample of this blood is labeled with Cr^{51} and injected into the patient. By periodically assaying for the radiolabel one can measure the rate of disappearance of the red cells. This permits the calculation of a red cell survival curve for the unit in question. If the computed survival is within normal limits, the transfusion can be given with confidence. On the other hand, drastically reduced survival indicates possible immune clearance and the transfusion of such donor blood could result in a hemolytic transfusion reaction.[3]

SPECIAL CASES

Donor selection and cross-match for patients who have received blood in the recent past that was other than their own group (universal donor and/or universal recipient), fetuses, newborn infants, and babies less than three months of age are cases that must be given special consideration.

The sera of patients who have received universal donor blood may contain traces of anti-A and anti-B. The concentration of these antibodies may equilibrate at substantial levels if more than a single unit of such blood was administered. Thus the group A patient who received several units of group O blood during a recently arrested acute bleeding episode may exhibit free anti-A antibodies in addition to the expected anti-B. A state of equilibrium exists in the patient with respect to these antibodies and the total antigen concentration and as such may result either in no effect or in a somewhat shortened survival of the patient's own red cells. However, under the conditions of a subsequent transfusion of group-specific blood (in this case group A blood), the equilibrium is disturbed and the free antibodies can attack the infused cells, resulting in a hemolytic episode.

Therefore, patients who have received blood other than their own group during a particular course of transfusion therapy should subsequently continue to receive blood of that group during the entire episode. Only when their cross-matches are completely nonreactive with blood of their own group can group-specific blood be administered.

Individuals less than three months of age, including fetuses and newborns, have little of their own alloantibodies, since humans do not begin to display the production of such antibodies until age three months. However, their sera contain maternal antibodies that have been acquired in intrauterine life by transplacental passage. Therefore, the most representative example of the antibody content of an infant's plasma is given by the maternal serum. Consequently, all cross-matches for the transfusion of babies who have never been transfused and who fall into this age group should be performed with the serum of the mother rather than the serum of the baby if this is at all possible.

Mothers do not always share major blood groups with their infants. It is possible for a group O mother to have a group A baby and vice versa. In view of these circumstances the ABO blood group selected for the transfusion of a baby must always be compatible with that of the mother. Otherwise, a hemolytic transfusion reaction could result. For practical purposes it is usually best to select group O blood and administer it as packed cells.

Antibodies in the donor plasma reactive with the patient's cells are critical in these cases since the normal effects of dilution are not experienced because of the relatively small total blood volume of the infant.

TRANSFUSION REACTIONS

Transfusion reactions are classified into several types. Hemolytic transfusion reactions result from the interaction of antibodies in the recipient's serum with antigens present on the red cells of the donor. Febrile transfusion reactions are characterized by an abrupt elevation in body temperature and can be caused by bacterial pyrogens or, most often, the interaction of leukocyte antibodies with their specific antigens. The offending antibodies may be present in the serum of either the recipient or the donor. Allergic transfusion reactions are characterized by the appearance of hives and may be accompanied by asthmatic symptoms. These may be caused by a preexisting allergy to plasma proteins. Some of these reactions have been traced to the presence of anti-IgA antibodies.

Safe blood transfusion practices dictate that whenever the recipient of a blood transfusion experiences any distressing symptoms, the transfusion is to be stopped and all materials returned to the blood bank for investigation.

The specific procedures to be followed by the blood bank laboratory in investigating any type of transfusion reaction will vary somewhat, depending on the institution. However, there is some commonality in that they are all designed to rule out the possibility of a hemolytic reaction.

Apart from a urinalysis, plasma hemoglobin determination, and bacterial cultures, which are performed in other sections of the laboratory, the properly documented investigation of any suspected transfusion reaction is the sole responsibility of the director of the blood bank laboratory. The first step to be taken is to recheck all identification on the pilot tubes in the laboratory, the patient on floor, and the unit of blood that was implicated. The second step includes a direct antiglobulin test on the cells of the recipient collected immediately after the reaction was first noted. This will determine whether or not there are any antibody-coated cells still present in the recipient's circulation. Presumably these would be donor cells sensitized by recipient antibodies, and therefore would be present in relatively small numbers, giving only a weakly positive test. Finally, all blood group determinations and cross-matches are repeated not only on the original pilot sample in the laboratory but with fresh samples collected after the reaction as well as with the contents of the returned blood bag itself. These tests should be performed by a technologist other than the one who did the original testing.

If all of these tests prove negative, it can be assumed that the reaction was not a hemolytic one and transfusion therapy can be resumed with a different unit of blood.

Unless the laboratory is properly equipped, it is not possible to establish positively that the reaction was caused by white cell antibodies or an allergic phenomenon. However, if these are suspected it is wise to administer buffy-coat poor blood in the case of possible febrile reactions and packed red cells in the case of possible allergic reactions.

TESTS IN HEMOLYTIC DISEASE
OF THE NEWBORN

Diagnostic tests in hemolytic disease of the newborn can be divided into three categories: prenatal diagnosis, postnatal diagnosis, and tests associated with prophylactic measures. If hemolytic disease of the newborn is suspected, it is essential to establish its presence early in the pregnancy. The majority of damage to infants suffering from this disease results from the accumulation of excess bilirubin. This occurs late in gestation and shortly after delivery. In severe cases, profound anemia, even during intrauterine life, can be life-threatening.

All diagnostic tests begin with an extensive blood grouping of the mother and the father of the child, which should include an ascertainment of the possible Rh genotypes. Usually all $D(Rh_o)$ negative mothers with $D(Rh_o)$ positive husbands are suspect, since from 50 to 100% of the offspring of such matings will be $D(Rh_o)$ positive, depending on the genotype of the father. The determinants of these genotypes will help to establish these probabilities. During a first pregnancy with no history of blood transfusion, miscarriage, or abortion, little else is done in the early stages.

Toward the end of the first pregnancy it is often worthwhile to obtain serum for an antibody screen not only for anti-D but also for any other antibodies that might have been formed. This testing will provide an indication of a primary response and aid in decisions regarding prophylaxis that need to be made after delivery.

Since most of the ravaging effects of hemolytic disease of the newborn are experienced in the second and subsequent pregnancies, they are normally followed more closely. Initially, antibody screenings are performed to detect the onset of immunization in the mother. Once the presence of antibodies is detected and their specificity ascertained, antibody titrations may be performed at various intervals to judge antibody level and thus monitor the progress of the immunization.

Although the measurement of antibody level gives some indication of the extent of the maternal immune response, it gives little if any information about the clinical condition of the infant. To obtain direct information on the severity of alloantibody effects on the fetus, the clinician may elect to perform a more direct test, which consists of a sampling of the amniotic fluid.

This procedure, known as amniocentesis, has certain risks to both the mother and the child. Consequently, it is performed only when the benefits clearly outweigh the risks, as when there is an established history of severe hemolytic disease of the newborn, or a strong suspicion of its occurrence based on immunization history and antibody level. In no case should amniotic fluid analysis be considered a substitute for a good serologic work-up.

The amniotic fluid is normally tested for the presence and quantity of bilirubin pigment. Massive destruction of the infant's red cells due to maternal alloantibodies causes an accumulation of these pigments. By comparing the bilirubin level in the amniotic fluid at a given point during gestation with a series of standard curves, one can establish a prognosis for the intrauterine survival of the infant and the extent of its anemia.[8] Usually this procedure is repeated on several occasions and the results compared. According to these results, the clinician may elect to terminate the pregnancy if the infant is mature enough to survive extrauterine life or to treat the infant's anemia by transfusions given in utero.

During intrauterine life, the anemia of hemolytic disease of the newborn is the primary threatening factor, the bilirubin only secondary since it is normally metabolized by the maternal liver. This is in contrast to the situation after birth when the bilirubin is the primary danger. This pigment can not be readily metabolized by the infant's immature liver and accumulates to reach high levels.

Blood for intrauterine transfusion, when it is indicated, must be compatible with the serum of the mother. It is infused into the peritoneal cavity of the fetus as packed cells. Interestingly, these transfused red cells are readily absorbed from the infant's peritoneal space into the circulation. Cases severe enough to require this form of therapy frequently require more than one transfusion during the course of the pregnancy.

In all suspected cases of hemolytic disease of the newborn, i.e., D(Rh$_o$) negative mothers both with and without demonstrable antibodies, laboratory tests are performed on the infant's cord blood immediately after birth to ascertain the presence of the disease. These tests include a measurement of the hemoglobulin, the total red cell mass and morphology, and the bilirubin level. If the infant in question does have a hemolytic anemia, the hemoglobulin and hematocrit will be below normal levels, the bilirubin will be elevated, and the smear will show an inordinately large number of nucleated red cells or normoblasts (erythroblasts). The latter is a characteristic feature of the disease process and gave it its original name, *erythroblastosis fetalis.*

In the meantime, the blood bank laboratory will be called on to determine the infant's blood group and Rh type and to attempt to demonstrate the presence of antibodies on the red cell surface by the direct antiglobulin test. Since only IgG immunoglobulins possess the molecular structure required for transplacental transfer, the antibodies present on the infant's red cell will belong to this class. Because in most blood group systems IgG immunoglobulins are incomplete antibodies that fail to agglutinate red cells under normal circumstances, the antiglobulin test must be used. In this instance the test is said to be a direct test, since the red cells to be tested presumably have been already coated with antibodies in vivo. The direct antiglobulin test will be positive in the majority of cases of hemolytic disease of the newborn. If the test is positive the degree of agglutination observed should be reported, since this serves as a crude indicator of the amount of antibodies bound and hence the potential severity of the disease.

Infants suffering from uncomplicated hemolytic disease of the newborn due to an Rh incompatibility frequently appear normal at birth. Visible signs of jaundice may not become apparent for up to twenty-four hours postpartum. For this reason, laboratory tests are essential since a delay in instituting therapeutic measures can result in severe clinical consequences.

There is another form of hemolytic disease of the newborn that results from an ABO incompatibility between mother and child. This occurs most frequently when the mother is group O and the infant group A. In these cases the mothers can form an "immune" variety of anti-A that is of the IgG class, is present in high titer, binds complement, and crosses the placenta in sufficient concentration to attack the infant's red cells. These infants are usually jaundiced at birth, their red cells exhibit marked spherocytosis, and unless special procedures are employed their direct antiglobulin tests may be only weakly positive or even negative because of vagaries exhibited by this type of antibody.[9] Definite diagnosis in some cases can only be established by eluting the suspected antibody from the infant's cells and showing that it is indeed anti-A. Because of the frequency of group O and group A in the population this is the most common form of hemolytic disease of the newborn. Fortunately, it is not as severe as the Rh form, partly because of the natural absorption of the antibody by the fetal tissues. It is self limiting and frequently requires no therapy.

In cases of severe hemolytic disease of the newborn the accepted therapeutic modality is exchange transfusion. This procedure, performed as soon after birth as possible, involves simultaneous removal of aliquots of the infant's blood and their replacement with fresh whole blood devoid of the antigens against which the maternal antibodies are directed. When the procedure is carried out with a single unit of donor blood, it allows the exchange of approximately 85% of the infant's total blood volume and accomplishes three things: it removes damaged red cells and replaces them with ones lacking the antigens and therefore cannot be destroyed by the antibodies; it removes maternal antibodies, thereby arresting the further destruction of newly developing infantile erythrocytes; and, most importantly, it removes bilirubin. In very severe cases, the procedure must be repeated several times on separate occasions to adequately flush out bilirubin and antibodies and to supply the patient with an adequate number of functioning red cells.

Blood selected for exchange transfusion in cases of Rh_o incompatibility is usually group O and always D (Rh_o) negative. Before use it must be cross-matched with the serum of the mother and shown to be nonreactive.

PROPHYLAXIS OF RH HEMOLYTIC DISEASE OF THE NEWBORN

Not long after hemolytic disease of the newborn was established as a clinical entity and its pathology explained in terms of maternal alloimmunization, it became clear that the frequency of Rh immunization was lower in those mothers who were ABO incompatible. It seems as if ABO incompatibility had some protective effect. One of the explanations proposed that in the situation of the group O, D (Rh_o) negative mother carrying a group A, D (Rh_o) positive fetus, the naturally occurring anti-A antibodies in the maternal plasma destroyed fetal group A, D (Rh_o) positive cells immediately on their entrance into the circulation. Presumably this destruction occurred rapidly enough to preclude an adequate interval for the initiation of immunization to Rh. This fact, coupled with the finding that the major stimulating dose of D (Rh_o) positive fetal cells is given to the mother as a result of the trauma of parturition, led to the development of the current prophylactic therapy.

Obviously the most frequent immunized mothers were those who were compatible with their fetuses with respect to ABO, making anti-A and anti-B useless as passively administered prophylactic agents. Nevertheless, since all of the mothers who have the potential to develop Rh antibodies are D (Rh_o) negative and their fetuses D (Rh_o) positive, a special type of anti-D antibody could be used for the same purpose. At present a commercial preparation of purified D (Rh_o) immune globulin is used for this purpose.[10] This preparation is designed to prevent primary immunization by masking or in some other way interfering with the immunogenecity of the D (Rh_o) antigen. Since primary immunization occurs most frequently as a result of the trauma of parturition during the course of the delivery, the immune globulin is given within seventy-two hours of this event.

Several laboratory tests are normally performed to ensure the efficacy of this substance. First, since treatment prevents immunization to only the D (Rh_o) antigen, it is customary to ascertain that the mother is truly D (Rh_o) negative and the infant is D (Rh_o) positive. Second, since the material will protect only against a primary response, if the mother has already been immunized, as evidenced by the presence of anti-D in her serum or a positive direct antiglobulin reaction is obtained with the infant's cells, the use of this material will be ineffectual. Finally, tests must be performed to ensure that an adequate amount of immune globulin is administered.

The Rh_o immune globulin preparation as supplied contains enough antibodies in a single dose to protect against immunization with up to 15 ml of packed fetal red cells. This is more than the normal volume of fetal red cells usually found in the maternal circulation as the result of the trauma of parturition. On cerain occasions however, the fetomaternal bleed may be greater, especially in cases of difficult delivery.

Several tests can be performed to determine the extent of fetomaternal bleed and therefore the dose of Rh_o immune globulin to be administered. First, each lot of immune globulin is accompanied by a test vial of material diluted in such a fashion that it will give no visible reaction with a sample maternal peripheral blood when a cross-match is done by the antiglobulin technique. On the other hand, if the level of fetal cells exceeds that capable of being rendered antigenically inactive by the standard dose of immune globulin, the cross-match will be positive.

A second method is designed to measure directly and more accurately the amount of fetal cells, such as the Kleinhaur-Betke acid elution technique for fetal hemoglobulin.[11] This is a special stain that can be performed on a smear of the mother's peripheral blood. The use of this stain allows the fetal red cells to be distinguished from the adult red cells. Therefore, it is possible to enumerate the fetal cells and accurately compute the value of fetomaternal bleed and the required dose of Rh_o immune globulin.

Rh immunization can occur whenever the D (Rh_o) negative mother is exposed to D (Rh_o) positive fetal cells, regardless of the outcome of the pregnancy. For this reason it is customary to administer Rh_o immune globulin to D (Rh_o) negative mothers who experience abortions and miscarriages in addition to deliveries of viable infants.

In summary, diagnostic tests performed in the blood bank laboratory fall into two broad categories: blood group antigen determination and blood group antibody detection. Safe blood transfusion demands a judicious use of both of these methodologies to match the donor and recipient for the major blood group and to ascertain that no harmful antibodies are present in the serum of either party. However, no degree of technical expertise will protect against a potentially dangerous transfusion reaction unless strict rules of clerical accuracy are maintained.

Tests for the detection of blood group antibodies are employed for the diagnosis of acquired hemolytic anemia. This may be of the alloantibody type, as exemplified by hemolytic disease of the newborn, or it may be of the autoantibody type, in which patients develop antibodies to their red cell antigens for no apparent reason. In each of these cases tests are performed for the presence of free antibodies in the serum and demonstrable by the indirect antiglobulin test, as well as for antibodies already bound to the erythrocytes and demonstrable by the direct antiglobulin test.

There are a number of acceptable methods for performing these procedures. Some of these methods are outlined in the appendices as a guide. However, the standard operating procedures pertaining to a given laboratory should be consulted for those methods approved by the laboratory director.

Review Questions

1. What is the most sensitive and practical screening test for fetomaternal bleeds?
2. A patient has three serum antibodies: anti-K, anti-Fy^a, anti-Jk^a. The antigen frequencies are: $K = 0.90$, $Fy^a = 0.65$, $Jk^a = 0.75$. What percentage of ABO group-specific blood would you expect to be compatible?
3. What type of donor would you select for a patient with anti-Hr″?
4. What is the optimum temperature for performing ABO grouping tests?
5. What is a possible explanation if the compatibility test is positive and the antibody screening test is negative?
6. When a blood specimen is grouped the following reactions are obtained.

ANTISERA			REAGENT CELLS		
A	B	A, B	A	B	O
+w	++++	++++	+w	o	o

What is the most likely explanation for these reactions?
7. What will most likely result from a transfusion of 100 ml of Group A blood to a Group O patient?
8. What usually is the specificity of cold autoagglutinins?
9. Group AB blood is needed for a severly anemic patient. There is none available; therefore, what would be the best blood to use?
10. What does the term transfusion reaction describe?
11. In Rh typing, what *must* one do?
12. What must the records of the evaluation of a transfusion reaction include?
13. What is the probable indentity of an antibody that reacts with the screening cells at room temperature only?
14. A newborn is Group O, Rh_o-positive and has a strongly positive direct antiglobulin test. The mother's antibody detection test is negative. Assuming the antibody detection is valid, what should be considered?
15. What is the most important antiserum used in doing an Rh typing?
16. What usually is the result of the direct antiglobulin test on the cord red cells of an infant affected with ABO hemolytic disease of the newborn?
17. A patient has autoimmune hemolytic anemia of life-threatening degree due to warm autoantibodies. All units cross-matched are incompatible; the auto control is strongly positive. What should the medical director do?

18. When a patient's blood is grouped with known sera and known cells, the following reactions are obtained:

ANTISERA			REAGENT CELLS		
A	B	A, B	A	B	O
++++	o	++++	o	o	o

What would the most likely explanation be?

19. You have been requested to supply blood for an exchange transfusion of a newborn with a tentative diagnosis of hemolytic disease of the newborn. The mother is group O, D (Rh$_o$) positive, the baby is group A, D (Rh$_o$) positive, and the direct antiglobulin test on the baby's blood was reported as +++. Three group O, D (Rh$_o$) negative and ten group O, D (Rh$_o$) positive donor units were cross-matched. Only one of the group O, D (Rh$_o$) positive units was found to be compatible. What is the most likely antibody in the mother's serum responsible for this problem?

20. An Rh$_o$-negative mother is known to be immunized to the D antigen. She delivers a baby who is typed as D (Rh$_o$) negative. The baby's direct antiglobulin test is ++++, cord bilirubin, 3.7 mg%, and the cord hemoglobin, 10.5 gm%. What is the most probable diagnosis of the baby's disease?

21. What is the mother's group if her two-day-old baby groups as O and his serum contains only anti-B?

REFERENCES

1. Ottenberg R: Studies in isoagglutination. I. Transfusion and the question of intravascular agglutination. J Exp Med 13:425, 1911.
2. Denis J: A letter concerning a new way of curing sundry diseases of transfusion of blood. Philos Trans R Soc Lond [Biol] 2:489, 1667.
3. Mollison PL: Blood Transfusion in Clinical Medicine. 6th ed. Oxford, Blackwell, 1979.
4. American Association of Blood Banks, Committee on Standards: Standards for Blood Banks and Transfusion Services. 10th ed. Washington, DC, AABB, 1981.
5. Morgan P and Bossom EL: "Naturally occurring" anti-Kell (K1): two examples. Transfusion 3:397, 1963.
6. Bowman HS, Brason FW, Mohn JF, and Lambert RM: Experimental transfusion of donor plasma containing blood-group antibodies into compatible normal human recipients. II. Induction of isoimmune haemolytic anemia by transfusion of plasma containing exceptional anti-CD antibodies. Br J Haematol 7:130, 1961.
7. Andrews AT, Zmijewski CM, Bowman HS, and Reihart J: Transfusion reaction with pulmonary infiltration associated with HL-A-specific leukocyte antibodies. Am J Clin Pathol 66:483, 1976.

8. Liley AW: Liquor amnii analysis in management of pregnancy complicated by rhesus sensitization. Am J Obstet Gynecol 82:1359, 1961.
9. Witebsky E: Interrelationship between the Rh and the ABO system. Blood 3:66, 1948.
10. Freda VJ, Robertson JG, and Gorman JG: Antepartum management and prevention of Rh isoimmunization. Ann NY Acad Sci 127:909, 1965.
11. Clayton EM Jr, Foster EB, and Clayton EP: New stain for fetal erythrocytes in peripheral blood stains. Obstet Gynecol 35:642, 1970.

CHAPTER 7

White Cell and Platelet Antigens and Antibodies

Objectives

In reading this section the student should learn the:

1. Alloantigens unique to certain formed elements of the blood apart from red cells.
2. Meaning of HLA and its clinical relevance.
3. Genetics and nomenclature of the HLA system.
4. Difference between Class I and Class II MHC antigens.
5. Problems associated with serologic cross-reactivity in the HLA system.
6. Principles of the cytotoxicity test.
7. Significance of granulocyte antigens and antibodies.
8. Problems associated with antibodies that react with antigens adsorbed into red cell membranes.

The term *blood groups,* according to present usage, refers to antigenic polymorphisms among humans that for the most part are confined to the erythrocytes. Although some of these antigens, such as A, B, and H, may also be found on other cellular components of the body, alloantigens representing the majority of blood group systems, such as Rh, Kell, Duffy, and so forth, are unique, antigenic characteristics of the red blood cells. By the same token, alloantigenic characteristics are present on the surface of leukocytes that are not found on red cells. Collectively these are referred to as leukocyte alloantigens, even though their occurrence is not restricted exclusively to the surface of white cells, some of them being present on platelets and nonhematopoietic nucleated cells of the body as well.

Apart from the rather widely distributed antigens of this group, certain specific alloantigens exist that are manifest only on individual members of the leukocyte series such as neutrophils, or subsets of lymphocytes and monocytes.

The importance of the leukocyte antigens has become increasingly apparent over the years in a number of contexts directly related to clinical laboratory practice. First, because of their presence on tissues and solid organs other than leukocytes, they have been considered as possible determinants of histocompatibility for organ transplantation. As such, they are frequently referred to as histocompatibility antigens, and organ donor-recipient matching is performed on this basis.

Second, antibodies to white cell antigens are frequently produced as a result of normal pregnancy as well as long-term whole blood or blood component transfusion. Therefore, knowledge of the leukocyte antigens and their antibodies is important in addressing the needs of people who depend on regular transfusions for the sustenance of life. Moreover, since some of the antigens to be discussed in this section are also found on platelets, antibodies to them can affect platelet survival. Therefore, these antigens in particular must be considered when transfusions of this blood component are used therapeutically.[1]

Third, since these alloantigenic characteristics, like those found principally on red cells, are under genetic control, they offer a completely different set of markers for the study of human genetics. They have achieved a prominent position in the determination of disputed paternity, in anthropologic investigations, and in investigations concerning their linkage with susceptibility to various human diseases that display familial tendencies.[2]

Finally, it has been shown that many of the products of the genetic complex controlling the production of a number of these antigens are an integral part of the chain of events leading to the immune response itself.[3] Indeed, some of the alloantigens controlled by this super locus and expressed on lymphoid cells form the basis of an intercellular communication network through which the immume system can be activated appropriately upon encountering antigens. Thus for the first time we are in the position of studying an alloantigenic blood cell system that has a specific biologic function.

The most readily recognized leukocyte and platelet antigens that are clinically relevant to blood transfusion and transplantation are those belonging to the HLA (*human leukocyte antigen*) system, which is a highly complex system of closely linked loci with multiple alleles whose genetics are somewhat comparable to those of the Rh blood group system.

THE HLA SYSTEM

HLA is probably the most polymorphic genetic system in humans. There are at least four serologically important loci in HLA, and a fifth controlling gene products that can be detected only in functional terms. The system contains over sixty distinguishable alleles, resulting in over 300,000 *haplotypes,* i.e., the combination of alleles from the separate loci occurring on a single chromosome. Extrapolating this number to the population results in well over ninety million possible phenotypes. Considering only the frequency of the major alleles in the population, only one in 10,000 random individuals are compatible, i.e., only one in 10,000 random donors would have no antigens that were lacking in a given recipient.

The HLA complex or super locus is located on the distal third of the short arm of chromosome 6 and is known as the human *major histocompatibility complex* or MHC (Fig. 1). The immediate environs of the MHC comprise a highly complex genetic region that controls a number of functions having basic immunologic importance. It has been shown that comparable MHC regions are found throughout the animal kingdom. So far the complex has been studied in mice, rats, rabbits, dogs, chickens, guinea pigs, cows, horses, and various species of primates. The MHC regions of each of these species show striking analogies to one another. Even though different chromosomes are responsible in each of the species, the MHC of each species contains loci that have control over more or less identical biologic functions. In the lower animals, where selective breeding can be done, a region governing the control of the immune response has been identified within the major histocompatibility complex.[4] In view of the proven analogies that have been observed, there is no reason to believe that a comparable locus does not exist within the major histocompatibility complex of humans. It is apparent that the alleles found on human chro-

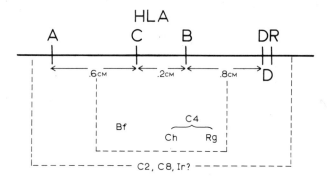

Fig. 1. A diagram of a segment of the distal third of the short arm of chromosome 6 carrying the HLA region referred to as the major histocompatibility complex. The centromere is located to the far right. In addition to bearing the HLA-A, B, C, and D-DR loci, the region also codes for the Properdin factor Bf and the C4 subcomponents Chido and Rodgers. In addition, evidence is available indicating that the region also contains loci controlling the complement components C2 and C8 as well as the hypothetical immune response genes, IR. Distances are expressed as centi-Morgans. (*After Amos.*[3])

mosome 6 exert a significant degree of influence on immunologic behavior, including self recognition and surveillance; thus the chromosome has been labeled by
some as one of the most biologically important chromosomes in humans.

GENETICS OF HLA

The HLA system is composed of five closely linked loci with corresponding independently segregating series of multiple allelomorphic genes. These in turn are responsible for the production of the various antigens (Table 1).

The arrangement of A, C, B, D, and DR loci situated on the chromosome is
such that the A and B loci are further apart than B and C. C is located between A
and B. D and DR are found as far away from B as is A so that B is actually between
and equidistant from A and D, DR. Although these loci are closely linked, recombination can occur with a frequency of 0.8% between A and B and between B and D.

The antigenic products of the A, B, and C locus alleles, referred to as Class I
MHC determinants, are membrane antigens present on all nucleated cells as well as
platelets. In addition, they are readily detected serologically by the microlymphocytotoxicity test. This test involves the interaction of specific antibodies with surface
antigens on lymphocytes, which activates complement and results in cell death. It
will be discussed in detail further on in this chapter. Chemically, Class I antigens
are composed of two polypeptide chains. The larger of the chains is about 44,000
daltons, contains a trace amount of carbohydrate and is slightly different for each of
the antigens in terms of only a few amino acids in its sequence. The smaller chain is
12,000 daltons and identical to β_2-microglobulin. This chain is constant among all
Class I antigens. In contrast, the antigens of the D series, called Class II MHC determinants, have a limited distribution and do not contain β_2-microglobulin as part
of their polypeptide structure. They are found primarily on B-lymphocytes, immunologically activated T-cells, macrophages, endothelial cells, and certain other specialized cell types. They can only be detected by means of the mixed lymphocyte
culture reaction (MLC or MLR) (Fig. 2). This is a test in which lymphocyte populations from two different individuals are mixed and incubated with each other in
tissue culture. Under such conditions, one population of cells (responders) will recognize any antigenic disparity for HLA-D on the second population of cells (stimu-
lators), which have been previously rendered immunologically nonreactive with
metabolic inhibitors such as mitomycin-C or X-ray. Having recognized the HLA-D
difference, the responders will undergo blastogenic transformation, which can be
measured.

The HLA-D antigens are of little importance in blood transfusion and any in-
depth consideration of their significance or the details used for their detection is beyond the scope of this work.

The antigens resulting from genes of the DR locus are classified as Class II
MHC determinants as well, and, like the HLA-D antigens, have a limited distribu-
tion confined primarily to B-lymphocytes, monocytes, endothelial cells, activated
T-cells, and certain other specialized cells. However, unlike the HLA-D antigens,

TABLE 1. THE RECOGNIZED HLA ALLELES

Locus A	Locus B	Locus C	Locus D	Locus DR
A1	B5	Cw1	Dw1	DR1
A2	Bw51*	Cw2	Dw2	DR2
A3	Bw52*	Cw3	Dw3	DR3
A9	B7†	Cw4	Dw4	DR4
Aw23	B8†	Cw5	Dw5	DR5
Aw24	B12	Cw6	Dw6	DRw6
A10	Bw44*	Cw7	Dw7	DR7
A25	Bw45†	Cw8	Dw8	DRw8
A26	B13*		Dw9	DRw9
Aw34	B14†		Dw10	DRw10
A11	B15		Dw11	
A28	Bw62†		Dw12	
A29	Bw63*			
Aw30	B16			
Aw31	Bw38*			
Aw32	Bw39†			
Aw33	B17			
Aw36	Bw57†			
Aw43	Bw58*			
	B18			
	Bw21			
	Bw49*			
	Bw50†			
	Bw22			
	Bw54†			
	Bw55†			
	Bw56†			
	B27*			
	Bw35†			
	B37*			
	B40			
	Bw60†			
	Bw61†			
	Bw41†			
	Bw42†			
	Bw46†			
	Bw47*			
	Bw48†			
	Bw53*			
	Bw59*			

*Bw4 Associated (See Text)
†Bw6 Associated (See Text)

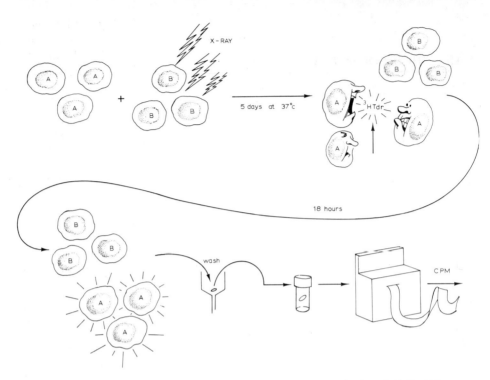

Fig. 2. The principle of the mixed lymphocyte culture reaction (MLC). When a population of lymphocytes, A, recognizes foreign HLA-D antigens on the surface of a second population of lymphocytes, B, the individual cells respond by undergoing blastogenic transformation. The population bearing the foreign antigen is pretreated with X-ray to render it incapable of responding itself. Therefore, all blastogenic transformation can be attributed to the responding cells. DNA synthesis occurs during this event and can be measured by feeding the cells a radiolabeled DNA precursor.

the DR antigens can be detected easily with specific antibodies in the microlymphocytotoxicity test.

When the DR antigens were first discovered, it was believed that they were the serologic counterpart of the MLC detectable HLA-D. Since then it has been shown that this is not the case. These antigens are somewhat similar in their cell distribution and behavior to the mouse IA antigens that have some bearing on immune responsiveness in that species. Apart from their potential usefulness as investigational probes into immune responsiveness and association with certain diseases in humans and their importance in organ transplantation, the DR antigens have little or no known practical application to blood transfusion at this time.

The nomenclature used in the HLA system is worthy of a special note. Each antigen carries a name composed of a letter A, B, C, D, or DR followed by a number sometimes accompanied by the prefix w. The letter refers to the specific HLA locus that controls the production of the antigen. The number refers to the specific allele and is assigned by the nomenclature committee of the World Health Organization when it is satisfied that a newly proposed leukocyte antigen is unique and can also be shown to be under the genetic control of the HLA system. Until these criteria are fulfilled the antigen carries a temporary designation, which consists of a unique number with a w prefix standing for "workshop."[5]

The alleles of each of the HLA loci are mutually exclusive according to genetic definition. No more than one allele from each series is ever found on a single chromosome. Therefore, every individual exhibits the products of not more than two HLA alleles from each series, one from each of the parental chromosomes. Thus every person can have a maximum total of eight recognizable HLA antigens, six that can be detected serologically and two that can be determined only by means of the MLC.

For example, the antigenic determinants HLA-A1, A2, A3, A9, A10, and A11 are alleles of the HLA-A locus. Any individual can have only two of these since they are controlled by a single locus and are mutually exclusive; therefore, people may be HLA-A1, A2, HLA-A1, A3, or HLA-A2, A9, but never HLA-A1, A2, A9. This can be readily understood by drawing a direct analogy to the MNSs system, in which the M and the S may be considered closely linked loci within the system. Even though numerous alleles of M can be found, such as M^1, N, N^2, M^g, and so on, any given individual has only two of these and never more. The antigenic determinants inherited from a single parent make up one half of an individual's phenotype and are called a haplotype (Fig. 3). For example, there can be two individuals with the phenotype HLA-A1, 3, B7, 5. However, one might have haplotypes HLA-A1, B7/A3, B5, whereas the other will possess HLA-A1, B5/A3, B7. Such haplotype designations can only be deduced from family studies and are not performed except in very special cases.

In routine clinical practice such as that encountered in blood banking, only the antigens of the A and the B series are usually considered. One of the reasons for this is the lack of suitable reagents for the positive identification of antigens controlled by the C locus. Also, studies have shown that the HLA-C antigens are relatively poor immunogens that do not play a significant role in platelet transfusion.

When one is typing only for the antigens of the A and B series of alleles it is common to find people with four fully detectable antigens. Such people are said to carry a "full house" and are the only ones whose HLA types can be considered ac-

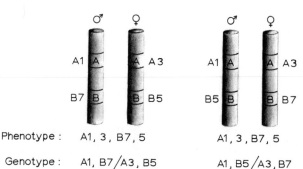

Phenotype :   A1, 3, B7, 5   A1, 3, B7, 5

Genotype :   A1, B7/A3, B5   A1, B5/A3, B7

Fig. 3. A diagrammatic representation of how the same phenotype can result from the expression of two different genotypes. The symbols refer to the parental origin of each MHC-bearing chromosomal segment.

curate within the limits of any biological test.

On occasion one may find people who lack a complete complement of HLA antigens. This apparently incomplete phenotype can be due to homozygosity for a given allele or to the presence of an allele whose expression cannot be detected because of the lack of appropriate antisera. People who carry less than four antigens are suspect unless homozygosity can be proved, since, because of the relative adolescence of the HLA typing science, one must always consider the existence of as yet undiscovered antigens.

In addition to the close linkage of the HLA loci, another relationship exists between certain individual alleles of the different loci. Under usual circumstances, if one is given two series of independent events, such as the alleles of the A and B series, one would expect to find a random assortment of pairs in the population as a whole. Thus, for example, in any paired set of haplotypes expressing HLA-A1 we should find B5 or any of the other B series alleles with a probability in proportion to their gene frequency in the population. This is the normal state of affairs and the system as a whole is said to be in a state of equilibrium. However, this is not what is found when large populations are studied with respect to HLA. Certain combinations of A and B series antigens are found together more often than might be expected due to chance alone. This is especially true of HLA-A, B8 and HLA-A3, B7, which are frequently found together on one chromosome in the majority of populations examined. Further, it is not uncommon to find certain DR locus antigens in association with certain B locus antigens and certain B locus antigens in association with certain C locus antigens. Some of the more prominent gametic associations that are known to exist in this system are given in Table 2. This strikingly habitual association is known as linkage disequilibrium and was referred to in Chapter 5. It is a characteristic feature of the entire HLA system. As a matter of fact, some people have concluded that the frequent disease associations found in HLA may really be

TABLE 2. PROMINENT GAMETIC ASSOCIATIONS FOUND IN HLA[16]

Whites	Blacks
A1, B8	A29, B7
Aw30, B13	Aw30, Bw42
Aw33, B14	A29, Bw44
A3, B7	Aw23, Bw45
A25, B18	A2, Bw51
Aw23, Bw49	A3, Bw35
A11, Bw55	
A2, Bw44	
A29, Bw44	
B27, DR1	
B7, DR2	
B8, DR3	
B8, DR4	
B18, DR5	
B13, DR7	

due to the existence of potentially dangerous susceptibility genes that are in disequilibrium with HLA.

A measure of the linkage disequilibrium and therefore the gametic association is given by a factor called Δ, which is the difference between the observed haplotype frequencies and those expected by computing the product of the gene frequencies of the two alleles in the population. The value of Δ is directly proportional to the degree of disequilibrium so that the greater the Δ, the more significant the disequilibrium.

The gene frequencies of HLA alleles are distributed differently in different ethnic groups and among different races. This is reflected in a variation in frequencies of antigens and one of the major characteristics of the HLA system. The frequency distribution of representative antigens as they are found among different races is given in Table 3. This is another important feature of the system and lends itself to use in anthropologic studies. From a more practical point of view, it has to be taken into consideration when one is attempting to identify antibodies in patient sera. Any test cell panel used for this purpose should be composed of people of various racial origins, otherwise some of the specific antigens normally found in only one race or another can be missed.

Although the antigens of the HLA system are expressed on all nucleated cells, the bulk of the HLA antigens that are dealt with daily, the ones of the A and B loci, are most easily identified on small lymphocytes of both the T and B classes. Fortunately, small lymphocytes may be isolated with relative ease from the peripheral blood and lend themselves admirably to various serologic manipulations. Class I MHC antigens such as the products of the HLA-A and B locus alleles are detected by the lymphocytotoxicity test.[6] This is a serologic procedure that differs considerably from the agglutination test used in normal blood grouping.

THE CYTOTOXICITY TEST

This procedure, which had been in use by mouse immunogeneticists for a number of years, was adopted for the detection of HLA antigens after it had been shown that the agglutination technique on granulocytes employed by the early workers had certain limitations. Granulocytes normally are sticky cells, making them difficult to manipulate in serologic reactions. Furthermore, their expression of HLA is variable. Unfortunately, lymphocytes, which are more amenable to serologic manipulation, are not agglutinated by the alloantisera in normal use.

The lymphocytotoxicity test as currently used has been miniaturized so that exceedingly small volumes of reactants are required and its principle is actually quite simple (Fig. 4). Suspensions of isolated, viable peripheral blood lymphocytes are mixed with the appropriate antisera in the reaction wells of specially designed plastic plates (Fig. 5) and the plates incubated, usually at room temperature. During this time the antibody molecules become attached to the HLA antigens on the cell surface. After the initial binding phase has taken place, normal rabbit serum is added as a source of complement. The antigen-antibody complexes at the cell sur-

TABLE 3. HLA ANTIGEN FREQUENCIES IN VARIOUS POPULATIONS[16]

Antigen	American Whites	American Blacks	Japanese
HLA-A1	25.3	6.5	1.1
A2	47.4	29.6	43.2
A3	26.9	17.7	1.1
Aw23(9)	5.2	24.2	1.1
Aw24(9)	13.2	3.2	58.5
A25	4.2	1.6	0.1
A26	7.0	6.5	6.4
A11	12.0	1.6	17.2
A28	10.0	11.8	1.1
A29	7.3	12.4	0.4
Aw30	4.8	21.0	0.3
Aw31	6.5	7.5	15.3
Aw32	7.3	2.7	0.1
Aw33	2.8	9.7	13.1
Aw34	0.5	14.5	1.9
Aw36	0.4	2.7	0.5
Aw43	0.2	0.5	0.0
HLA-B7	19.3	14.7	11.4
B8	17.5	4.4	0.2
B13	5.2	2.2	4.0
B14	9.2	7.6	0.2
B18	9.1	8.2	0.0
B27	7.5	2.7	0.8
Bw35	15.1	14.1	14.1
B37	3.3	1.1	1.1
Bw38(w16)	6.6	0.0	0.4
Bw39(w16)	4.2	1.1	5.7
Bw41	3.2	1.6	0.7
Bw42	0.7	12.5	1.2
Bw44(12)	26.2	14.1	12.5
Bw45(12)	1.4	9.2	0.3
Bw47	0.5	0.0	0.4
Bw48	1.3	2.2	4.6
Bw49(w21)	5.1	7.1	0.6
Bw50(w21)	2.3	2.2	0.0
Bw51(5)	9.2	3.3	15.9
Bw52(5)	2.9	1.6	20.5
Bw53	0.2	16.9	0.2
Bw54(w22)	0.0	0.0	14.1
Bw55(w22)	3.9	1.1	5.8
Bw56(w22)	1.2	0.0	2.2
Bw57(17)	7.3	7.6	0.0
Bw58(17)	2.1	14.7	1.7
Bw59	0.9	2.0	4.2
Bw60(40)	11.9	3.8	12.7
Bw61(40)	2.3	1.6	16.8
Bw62(15)	9.7	1.6	16.7
Bw63(15)	2.0	0.5	0.4

TABLE 3. (Continued)

Antigen	American Whites	American Blacks	Japanese
HLA-Cw1	6.5	1.1	32.1
Cw2	8.6	17.9	0.7
Cw3	23.0	17.4	46.5
Cw4	19.6	30.4	9.3
Cw5	12.0	5.4	0.2
Cw6	14.4	13.6	1.4
Cw7	6.1	7.6	2.1
Cw8	4.7	1.1	0.2
HLA-DR1	20.4	13.7	12.2
DR2	26.3	33.9	36.0
DR3	22.7	28.0	3.2
DR4	28.0	8.3	41.4
DR5	18.8	29.2	4.3
DRw6	7.3	8.9	9.1
DR7	22.8	22.0	1.0
DRw8	5.9	12.5	12.6
DRw9	2.5	4.8	23.0
DRw10	0.7	1.8	1.2

face activate the complement, which then kills the cells. Cell death is ascertained by observing their morphology microscopically under conditions of phase contrast illumination after treatment with supra vital stains. Living and dead cells can be distinguished from each other because they possess different optical properties. In addition, living cells are able to actively eliminate certain intracellular dyes to which they are exposed, whereas dead cells do not have this capability. As a result, under the appropriate lighting conditions living cells appear as refractile, colorless, and compact, while dead cells are densely colored and swollen with prominent nuclear detail. A positive reaction indicative of the antigen-antibody reaction is ascertained by determining the percentage of dead cells. After some practice this can be judged by the overall microscopic appearance of the entire contents of the reaction well (Fig. 6).

Many different dyes are used to accentuate the morphological differences between living and dead lymphocytes. The two most common are eosin Y and trypan blue. Of the two, eosin Y is the easiest to use. It imparts an intense and very deep maroon color to dead cells, which then appear to be in sharp contrast against a very bright red background. On the other hand, living cells stained with the same dye glow bright yellow. Trypan blue stains dead cells a very pale blue while living cells remain colorless. Some workers have difficulty in distinguishing the dead cells against the pale blue background imparted by the dye. Undiluted complement should not be used in trypan blue tests, since high protein concentrations interfere with the uptake of this dye by the cells.

Since the end point of the cytotoxicity test is either a living lymphocyte or a dead lymphocyte, the preservation of the viability of the lymphocyte suspension is one of the most critical factors in all of the serologic tests associated with HLA. A

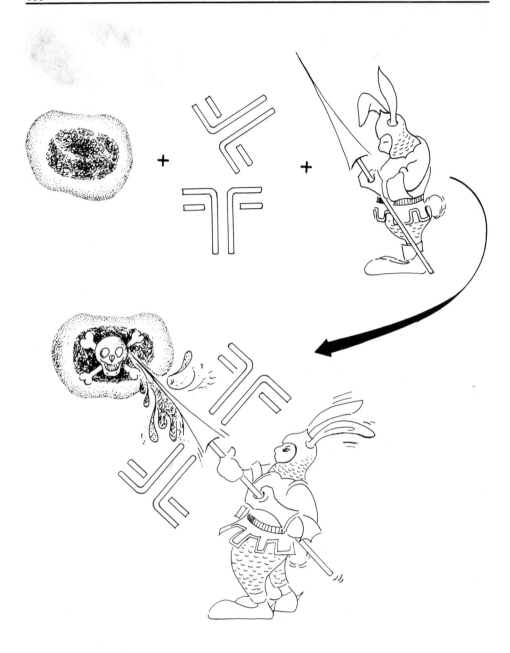

Fig. 4. This cartoon explains the basic principle of the cytotoxicity procedure. Viable lymphocytes express the HLA antigens on their surface. A suspension of these cells is mixed with appropriate antisera and two molecules of IgG antibody are bound to the antigens. This results in the activation of complement present in normal fresh rabbit serum. The activated complement kills the lymphocytes.

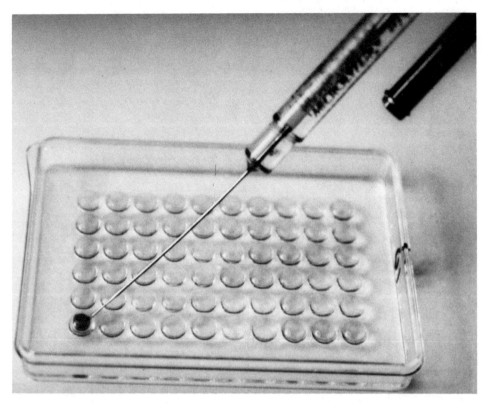

Fig. 5. A typical tray for use in the microlymphocytotoxicity test. The tray is 56 × 81 mm and fits on the stage of a microscope. It contains 60 wells that have optically flat bottoms in which the reactions take place. Each well is filled with mineral oil to retard the evaporation of the small volumes of reactants that are injected with a syringe designed for gas chromatography. The reactions are read through the bottom of the plate with an inverted microscope.

rudimentary knowledge of the properties of extracorporeal human small lymphocytes contributes greatly to providing a laboratory environment conducive to their optimal survival for testing purposes. After twenty-four hours in vitro, lymphocytes in whole blood begin to die at an extremely rapid rate. Therefore, if at all possible the tests should be performed on blood that is less than twenty-four hours old. If this is impossible for one reason or another, the cells should be separated and placed in a suitable nutrient tissue culture medium that contains appropriate antibiotics. Recipes are available for media that will support storage for up to five or six days. Also, lymphocytes appear to be extremely sensitive to changes in temperature. In the body these cells are maintained at 37C, but upon collection rapidly cool to room temperature. To avoid additional thermal shock it is best to store them at room temperature until they are ready for testing. Therefore samples for HLA typing should not be refrigerated. Storage at 37C should be avoided as well since this

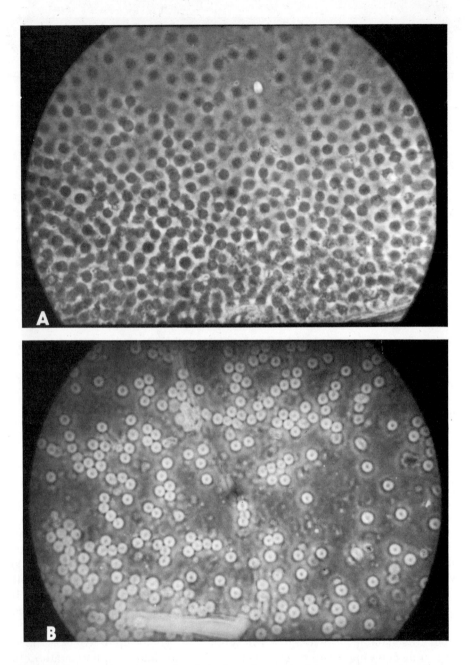

Fig. 6. Microscopic appearance of the lymphocytotoxicity reaction under phase contrast. **A.** A Positive Reaction. Almost all of the cells have taken up the dye. They are swollen with dense and prominent nuclear detail indicative of cell death. **B.** A Negative Reaction. The majority of cells are alive. They are of normal size, nuclear detail is all but absent, and the cells have a glistening appearance resulting from their ability to actively exclude the dye.

not only constitutes another temperature change but also can promote the growth of bacteria that may interfere with the normal resting state of the lymphocytes in a number of ways that are undesirable. Blood samples collected for lymphocyte separation should be collected in preservative-free (commonly used preservatives are toxic to lymphocytes) heparin as an anticoagulant or they may be defibrinated with glass beads. The cytotoxicity test is a complement-dependent procedure that requires Ca^{++} and Mg^{++} ions. Therefore, anticoagulants such as EDTA or ACD that chelate or bind heavy metals should be avoided.

The majority of antibodies associated with the HLA system are IgG immunoglobulins and the cytotoxicity reaction is complement-dependent. As previously discussed, for complement activation to occur, two molecules of IgG must be affixed to antigens on the cell surface in such a way that their Fc portions are in proximity. The ideal arrangement for this occurrence is when the antibodies combine with antigenic receptor sites that are adjacent to each other. One of the problems associated with HLA typing is the fact that the HLA molecules are not firmly affixed to the cell wall. Instead, they are anchored into the fluid lipid bilayer of the membrane by a small connecting piece but are otherwise floating freely on the cell surface. Thus, they can collect at various spots or disperse, depending on the conditions. These conditions may on occasion be dictated by the physiologic state of the individual being tested and ultimately may have some effect on the outcome of the serologic determinations. Therefore, appropriate positive and negative controls are absolutely essential.

Fresh, normal rabbit serum has been found to be the ideal source of complement for use in the lymphocytotoxicity test. One of the reasons for this is that normal rabbit serum contains trace quantities of naturally occurring antibodies against a human species-specific antigen. These antibodies tend to react synergistically with the HLA antibodies that are bound to their specific antigen by forming the bimolecular configuration required to bring about maximum complement activation. Not all examples of rabbit serum are a suitable source of complement. The sera of some rabbits may contain either too little complement or antihuman antibodies to be useful. The sera of other rabbits, on the other hand, may contain an excess of antihuman antibodies and are nonspecifically toxic to all cells. Therefore the rabbit serum used must be carefully screened and selected to give maximum specific killing with standard HLA antisera and at the same time have little or no cytotoxic activity of its own.

A peculiar phenomenon that is sometimes observed in cytotoxicity tests is one referred to as CYNAP. This stands for cytotoxicity negative absorption positive, which means that under certain circumstances a cell suspension from a particular individual will not be killed under the conditions of a cytotoxicity test even though it is capable of specifically binding the antibody and removing it from a serum by absorption. The lymphocytes of some individuals are more prone to exhibit this type of behavior than others. Similarly, certain sera are more prone than others to provoke this type of activity. The exact mechanism is unknown but a number of factors have been implicated as potential causes, including cellular abnormalities such as aberrant distribution of antigens at the cell surface that do not allow an orientation of antibody molecules that is appropriate to optimal complement activation, or nonspecific anticomplementary factors present in certain sera that lead to premature complement utilization.

Certain variations of the standard cytotoxicity procedure have been devised to minimize CYNAP reactions. One of these procedures, referred to as the Amos modified technique, includes a wash step performed immediately following the incubation with antibodies. During this step, most of the unbound serum proteins contributed by the antiserum are removed. The antibodies, since they are specifically bound, remain behind. Since most of the potentially anticomplementary factors encountered in the cytotoxicity system are "abnormal" proteins present in the antiserum used, the wash step minimizes anticomplementariness by removing interfering substances.

Another variation in technique is the antiglobulin cytotoxicity procedure.[7] As the name implies, a suitable antiglobulin serum is added to the cells that have been preincubated with antiserum and washed. This is subsequently followed by the addition of complement and a further incubation. This procedure either stabilizes the HLA antigen to anti-HLA complex on the cell wall or in some other way induces conformational changes that provide the appropriate molecular configuration for optimal complement binding. In this method, the choice of antiglobulin reagent as well as its concentration is critical and the particular reagent used must be carefully selected and standardized in each laboratory. It has been shown that antiglobulin reagents specific for immunoglobulin light chains are the sera of choice. Therefore sera commonly employed in the blood bank laboratory in the Coombs test are unsuitable for this purpose.

The use of either of these variations of the cytotoxicity procedure considerably increases the sensitivity of the reaction. This makes them extremely useful when attempting to detect the presence of antibody to HLA in an unknown serum. Very small amounts of antibodies will be detected even under the most adverse of circumstances. This same sensitivity, however, has a disadvantage in that it brings out a considerable degree of cross-reactivity (see below). Therefore, if they are employed in typing procedures using antisera whose specificity was ascertained by conventional methods, erroneous results will be obtained.

The sera used for the detection of HLA antigens are human alloantisera derived from two basic sources. The first of these is the patient accidentally immunized by transfusion or transplantation. Since the HLA antigens are expressed on leukocytes and platelets, patients who receive multiple blood transfusions are exposed to a continuous source of antigens. As a consequence of this exposure they produce HLA antibodies frequently. In addition, since the HLA antigens are human transplantation antigens by definition, patients who have received an organ transplant and subsequently reject their graft may display HLA antibodies in their sera.

Polytransfused patients are exposed to a large number of different HLA antigens from the variety of donors used in transfusion. Therefore, although such sera are of high titer and are potent cytotoxic agents, they tend to be multispecific and virtually useless as typing reagents. The sera of patients who have undergone organ transplantation, even though containing antibodies of more restricted specificity, as a result of the transplant, frequently contain additional antibodies produced as a result of pretransplant transfusions that may have been used in the treatment of their basic disease. Therefore, their sera are frequently multispecific as well and equally useless as typing reagents.[8]

The second and actually the primary source of HLA antisera used for clinical typing is the serum of multiparous women. Twenty-five percent of multipara (those who have had two or more pregnancies) have detectable anti-HLA antibodies in their sera. These antibodies are formed as a result of alloimmunization of pregnancy. Because under normal circumstances each pregnancy results in exposure to a limited number of separate HLA antigens of paternal origin, the chances of finding good, operationally monospecific reagents among these sera is very great.

Fortunately, even though HLA antibody production as a result of alloimmunization of pregnancy is common and results in the formation of IgG antibodies, it causes no ill effects as far as the infants are concerned. One of the possible reasons for this lack of pathologic effect is that the HLA antigens against which the antibodies are directed are adequately expressed in the cells of the placenta. Therefore, any antibodies that cross the placenta are trapped within the placental network. However, this does not apply to antibodies directed against granulocyte or platelet-specific antigens, which may cause harmful effects, as will be described later. A second reason may be that neonates have only low levels of complement and therefore a suitable effector mechanism is not in operation.

CROSS-REACTIVITY

Serologic cross-reactivity is not a new concept in immunology, but it is one that has not been discussed in any detail since it plays only a minor role in the elucidation of red cell antigens. This is not the case in the HLA system. Cross-reactivity in the context of HLA is a prominent feature and must be considered not only in the identification of antibodies but in the assignment of antigens to a given cell. For clarity and convenience this question is often approached from the point of view of the cross-reactivity of antisera even though the roots of the problem lie in the biochemical structure of the antigen.

The cross-reactivity of the antisera usually encountered in leukocyte grouping is a normal rather than an extraordinary event. It can be implicated whenever sera contain antibodies that can be shown to be reactive with more than one antigen and cannot be separated even with the most carefully designed analytical absorption procedures. This finding is somewhat analogous to the behavior of the anti-A, B found in group O sera or that of anti-M and anti-N produced in rabbits. Sera of this variety may be used as typing reagents if one resorts to certain serologic tricks, such as employing several examples of antiserum from different sources or performing comparative titrations, but this is not the most desirable approach. Nevertheless, this remains a major problem associated with both the selection of appropriate reagents for the determination of the HLA types and the interpretation of the final typing results. Fortunately, the distribution of the specificities in cross-reactive sera is such that extreme examples that could seriously compromise reliable typing are encountered infrequently. Therefore, under normal circumstances a selection of three or more sera identifying any of the more common specificities often gives interpretable results. However, because of the problem of cross-reactivity a single antiserum can never be used to ascertain even the most well-established of the HLA antigens.

Cross-reactivity is an important consideration when one is attempting to identify the specificity of an antibody in a given serum. In this connection, it is worthwhile to define some common terms often used in describing anti-HLA sera that imply cross-reactivity. Frequently, such reagents may be referred to as "long," "short," "broadly reactive," or "included." These terms are colloquialisms referring to histograms, the tools habitually used by workers in this field. A better understanding of their meaning can be obtained from Figure 7, which represents a portion of data collected in the first HLA Workshop of the Americas. In this example, sera 107 and 109 are "long" since they react with more cells than those that contain the reference antigen B5, while sera 098 and 270 are "short." Serum 089 might also be referred to as a "broadly reactive" or "supertypic" serum since it "includes" the reactions of sera 098 and 270 and encompasses the entirety of the reference antigen. Therefore, the pattern obtained when the reactions of certain sera are included within the scope of a broadly reactive serum may give the impression of being due

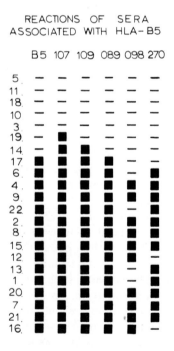

REACTIONS OF SERA
ASSOCIATED WITH HLA-B5

Fig. 7. A histogram formed from some of the data on anti-HLA-B5 sera from the first HLA Workshop of the Americas, showing "long" and "short" sera, as well as "inclusions."

— = NEGATIVE

■ = POSITIVE

TABLE 4. AN ILLUSTRATION OF CROSS-REACTIVITY DUE TO SHARED ANTIGENIC DETERMINANTS

HLA Specificity	Hypothetical Antigenic Determinant	Possible Antibodies Produced	Observed Antiserum Specificity	Reactions with:		
				B5	Bw35	B18
B5	A B C	anti-A anti-B anti-C	anti-B5	++	+	+
Bw35	A D E	anti-A anti-D anti-E	anti-Bw35	+	++	+
B18	C F E	anti-C anti-F anti-E	anti-B18	+	+	++

to the existence of subgroups. Although this is not really the case, the concept is a convenient way of illustrating the problem.

The cross-reactivity of antisera habitually observed is attributable directly to the cross-reactivity of the HLA antigens. The chemical analysis of the HLA fine structure has revealed only very minute differences between the various antigenic specificities studied to date. Thus it can be said that a considerable degree of homology between different HLA antigens exists at the molecular level. From this, it can be concluded that cross-reactions are observed most probably because of the existence of multiple shared antigenic determinants that result in the appearance of a variety of antibody specificities in any given antiserum. This is illustrated in Table 4.

The commonly encountered cross-reactive groups (CREGS) of HLA antigens can be arranged in clusters, as shown in Figure 8.[3] These cross-reactive groups must be taken into consideration when selecting HLA typing sera, assigning HLA antigens, and making decisions about "compatible" donor recipient pairs.

Apart from the CREGS yet another type of cross-reactivity exists among the antigens of the HLA-B series. This is imparted by the so-called supertypic antigens Bw4 and Bw6. These antigenic determinants apparently form a structure which is common to a group of HLA-B gene products. Consequently some of the antigens such as Bw51 and B13 are also Bw4, whereas others such as B7 and B8 are Bw6 (Table 1).

Generally speaking, antisera will be less cross-reactive if they come from donors who themselves possess one or more antigens of the cross-reactive groups. From the standpoint of discrimination, for example, the very best anti-HLA-B5 sera are produced by people who have the Bw35 antigen. These people, since they share the A antigenic determinant cited in Table 4, can only make anti-B and C. By the same token, such sera are produced infrequently since B5 is much less immunogenic when used to challenge a Bw35 individual than one who is lacking all the antigens of the cross-reactive group.

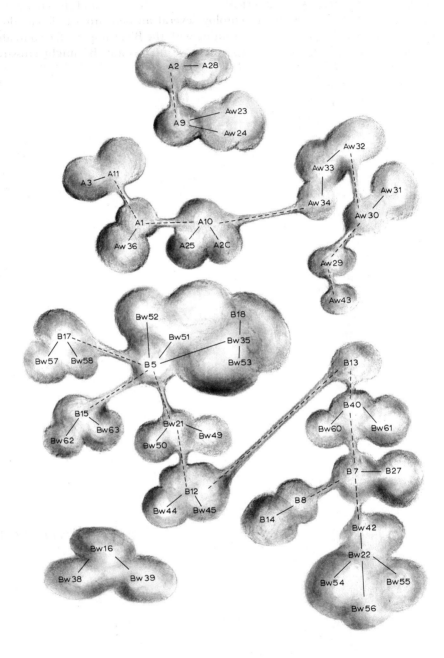

Fig. 8. Clusters of cross-reactive groups (CREGS) of the HLA antigens. Dotted lines represent weak or loose cross-reactivity.

To safeguard against the interference of cross-reactivity and the creation of a typing problem, it is necessary to employ several antisera from different donors directed against each specificity. Continuing with the B5 example referred to above and illustrated in Table 4, one antiserum classified as anti-B5 might cross-react with B5, Bw35, and B18, a second with B5 and Bw35, and a third with B5 and B18. A cell that reacts with all three of these sera can be said to have the antigen B5 since this is the only cross-reactive specificity that is shared by the three antisera.

According to the present state of the art, most workers engaged in routine clinical typing use approximately seventy different antisera to define very crudely the thirty most prevalent antigens of the A and B loci. For a more precise estimation of these antigens almost 100 sera are needed. Our knowledge of these cross-reactive groups has increased considerably since the early 1970s; it is hoped that reagents will be prepared in the future by newer technology that will clearly distinguish among the antigens of any given cross-reactive group.

To some degree the existence of the cross-reactive groups in the HLA system is beneficial. Because of the extensive polymorphism of the system, with its almost astronomical number of phenotypes, it is often difficult if not impossible to find donors of solid organs or blood components who are an exact match for a given recipient. Fortunately, in most cases the scheme of matching donors and recipients based on the sharing of cross-reactive groups is adequate and its use in some platelet programs yields good results.[9] According to this approach, a recipient of HLA type A9, 3, B12, 7 could receive platelets from a donor of type A9, 1, B12, 8 since A3 and A1 as well as B7 and B8 each belong to their own respective cross-reactive groups. Conversely it might be unwise to use a donor who is A9, 3, B5, B17, since B5 belongs to different cross-reactive groups than B12 and B7.

GRANULOCYTE-SPECIFIC ANTIGENS

In addition to the antigens of the HLA system, granulocytes express their own characteristic antigens. They may be detected by granulocyte agglutination, granulocyte cytotoxicity, or by indirect immunofluorescence tests using appropriate sera from multiparous women or from patients with certain diseases characterized by granulocytopenia. Originally three alloantigens restricted to neutrophilic granulocytes were described by Lalezari.[10] These have been designated NA_1, NA_2, and NB_1, and are presumably under the control of two genetically independent loci, NA and NB. A third allelic series, NC, was heralded by the discovery of the antigen NC_1.

In contrast to HLA antibodies formed during pregnancy that cause no harm to the fetus, anti-NA, NB, and NC antibodies produced in a similar fashion attack the fetal neutrophils. Presumably this can occur because the antibodies are not absorbed by placental tissue, which lacks the appropriate antigen. The antibody-mediated neutrophil destruction results in a disease known as neutropenia of the newborn. Infants suffering from this condition are born with a dangerously low granulocyte count that may persist for up to four to six weeks. Frequently the patients present a variety of severe bacterial infections that demand aggressive antibiotic therapy. Since once the condition occcurs in one infant it is almost certain to occur in the subsequent infants in a given family, antibiotics are sometimes given prophylactically. Fortunately, because of the high frequency and distribution of the antigens (Table 5) in the population, coupled with the fact that an immunizing dose of antigen can be delivered only by fetal neutrophils, appropriate conditions for alloimmunization of pregnancy do not occur very often. Therefore antibody formation is rare and the disease infrequent.

Since the original description of the NA, NB, and NC systems, two other neutrophil-specific antigens, ND_1 and NE_1, have been discovered by means of antisera found in patients suffering from autoimmune neutrophil granulocytopenia and chronic benign neutropenia, respectively. Supposedly these alleles are controlled by separate loci, but the appropriate linkage studies have not been performed. Interestingly, the gene frequency of NE_1 is 0.12, which is the postulated gene frequency of the missing allele of ND_1. It is entirely possible that NE_1 is really ND_2, but confirmation must await appropriate family studies.

Apart from the neutrophil-specific antigens other antigens appear to be represented on all members of the granulocytes series (see Table 5). The antigens of the 5 and 9 systems were discovered along with the antigens that now form the HLA system. Later they were shown to be independent of HLA and restricted to granulocytes and some additional nucleated cells of non-hematopoetic origin. They are defined with sera from normal multipara and do not appear to be associated with any pathologic conditions in the antibody producer or the offspring.

The antigens of the HGA series are defined with antibodies produced as a result of transfusion with either pure granulocyte components or granulocyte-contaminated platelet components. As such, they may prove to be of some significance in determining the success or failure of such therapeutic procedures.

In contrast to the N series antibodies, anti-NA, anti-NB, etc., which with but a single exception work well in agglutination tests, anti-HGA antibodies can be detected most reliably with a two-color fluorochromatic microgranulocytotoxicity assay. This is a variation of the standard cytotoxicity test in which granulocytes are substituted for lymphocytes as antigen bearing targets. The cells are prelabeled with a potentially fluorescent compound (fluorescein diacetate—broken down by intracellular enzymes into fluorescein) that escapes from the cell when it is damaged by complement. When such preparations are examined microscopically under ultraviolet light, the live cells glow with an apple-green fluorescence, while the dead cells are normally invisible since they do not contain the fluorescent dye. To help visualize the dead cells, the final reaction mixture is further stained with ethidium bromide. This dye gives off a red fluorescence under ultraviolet light and is excluded from live cells, but penetrates dead ones, staining their nuclei. Therefore, in the two-color assays live cells glow green and dead ones red.

Since antibodies to any of the antigens just described can destroy granulocytes in vivo with the release of both toxic and vasoactive substances, they have the ability to produce the classic form of febrile transfusion reaction under appropriate conditions. Reactions of this type resulting from sudden and massive granulocyte

TABLE 5. GRANULOCYTE ANTIGENS

Ag	Gene Frequency	Antigen Frequency (%)	Mode of Detection	Clinical Association	Reference
NA₁	0.377	61.9	Agglutination	Associated with granulocytopenia of the newborn and febrile transfusion	17
NA₂	0.633	87.7	Agglutination	"	17
NB₁	0.83	96.9	Agglutination	"	17
NC₁ (VAZ)	0.80	96.0	Agglutination		18
9ᵃ	0.345	57.1	Agglutination	Multipara	18
5ᵃ	0.200	36.0	Agglutination	Multipara	18
5ᵇ	0.800	96.0	Agglutination	Multipara	
ND₁	0.88	98.5	Indirect Immunofluorescence (only?) IgG and IgM	Autoimmune neutrophil granulocytopenia	19
NE₁(ND₂)	0.12	23.0	Agglutination	Chronic benign neutropenia	20
HGA-3a	0.1140	21.4	2-color fluorescent cytotoxicity or fluorochromatic microgranulocytotoxicity	Multiple transfusion including granulocyte transfusion	21
3b	0.1281	22.4			
3c	0.0842	16.03			
3d	0.3122	52.6			
3e	0.090	17.1			

destruction produce severe symptoms, which may include pulmonary edema and sometimes even death.[11]

In contrast to the hemolytic transfusion reaction that is most severe and clinically significant when it is associated with patient antibodies destroying donor cells, the white cell reaction can be equally severe when the antibodies are of donor origin. A possible reason for this is that the in vivo granulocyte antigen-bearing pool in the patient is much smaller than the red cell antigen-bearing pool. Therefore, a condition of antigen excess is not readily established. Furthermore, the antibodies involved are usually complement binding and are present in much higher concentrations than one would be led to believe by their in vitro titers. Therefore, antibody dilution alone affords little or no protection. In addition, at least one case of a severe reaction has been reported in which a potent antibody in the plasma of one donor reacted with the granulocytes in the fresh blood of a second donor. For these reasons, it is essential to take precautions when using blood donated by multipara who may have been immunized by pregnancy. Many institutions have adopted the policy of using such blood only in the form of packed red cells.

It should be noted in passing that the true febrile type of transfusion reaction is not restricted to antigen-antibody reactions within the granulocyte-specific systems. It can result with equal facility from the interaction of certain HLA antibodies that are directed against those particular HLA antigens that happen to be well-expressed on granulocytes. Among these are the HLA antigens originally discovered by the old method of EDTA agglutination on granulocytes and include HLA-A2 (MAC,8^a), B5 (part of 4^a), B7, B8, and B14 (all part of 4^b).

PLATELET-SPECIFIC ANTIGENS

The most notable platelet-specific antigen is $P1,^{A1}$, originally described by Shulman.[12] It has a frequency in the population of 97%, and therefore immunization is an infrequent event. However, individuals lacking $P1^{A1}$ may produce antibody after antigen challenge in the form of a transfusion or alloimmunization of pregnancy. Anti-$P1^{A1}$ antibodies, when they are found, react best by either complement fixation tests or an indirect radioimmune binding assay. In vivo the antibodies can cause rapid and catastrophic destruction of transfused platelets, leading to posttransfusion thrombocytopenic purpura, and when associated with pregnancy can result in thrombocytopenia of the newborn.

Occasionally the reaction of anti-$P1^{A1}$ in a recipient's serum with $P1^{A1}$ antigen or donor platelets can lead to destruction of the recipient's own platelets. This occurs through a poorly understood and highly speculative mechanism mimicking autoimmunity. Presumably the anti-$P1^{A1}$ produced cross-reacts with the patient's $P1^{A1}$ negative platelets. When this process occurs the patient's own platelets are rapidly destroyed as long as the antigen-incompatible platelets are being given. Frequently, though not always, the process may stop when the transfusion is terminated.

In view of the high frequency of this antigen in the population and its difficulty of detection, $P1^{A1}$ is not routinely considered in platelet transfusion.

WHITE CELL ANTIBODIES IN TRANSFUSION PRACTICE

Since the HLA antigens are well-developed on platelets, it is logical to assume that preimmunization against these antigens would have an adverse effect on platelet transfusion. As early as 1962 it was observed that decreased platelet survival was an exquisitely sensitive indicator of HLA immunization even in the apparent absence of demonstrable antibodies. With the increasingly popular use of platelet therapy it has become quite evident that this is the case. Even supposedly unimmunized recipients, after continuous platelet transfusion, become *refractory*. In other words, continued platelet infusion produces very little if any increment in the number of circulating platelets as well as no improvement in hemostasis.

The examination of sera from refractory patients usually reveals the presence of anti-HLA antibodies, and Yankee et al.[13] have shown that such patients could benefit from platelets that were HLA matched and therefore cross-match compatible. In addition, the use of HLA matched platelets from the outset of therapy can prevent the development of HLA antibodies and the onset of the refractory state in a fair proportion of patients.

The usefulness of HLA in improving the outcome of granulocyte transfusion has not been determined as yet, probably because granulocyte transfusions are not as common as platelet transfusions and the therapy, when it is instituted, is of short duration and usually is given to patients who are immunologically compromised for one or more reasons. Therefore, refractoriness as such has not become evident nor is it a real factor. The success or failure of granulocyte therapy is judged according to the clinical improvement of the patient in terms of warding off infection. There is no reason to suppose, however, that not only HLA but also the neutrophil antigens of the NA, NB, NC, ND, and NE series as well as the granulocyte antigens of HGA-3 will not gain some measure of significance as more experience is accumulated.

In the more routine blood transfusion service, antibodies to leukocyte antigens can be of significance for two reasons. First, they are the known causative agents of febrile transfusion reactions in polytransfused patients, multiparous women, and otherwise preimmunized individuals. Second, under certain circumstances they can agglutinate red cells in vitro and therefore interfere with the normal interpretation of red cell crossmatches by mimicking a true red cell incompatibility even though they do not cause decreased red cell survival of any other form of red cell destruction. Although most of the white cell antibodies detected in cases of febrile transfusion reactions are most frequently leukagglutinins with no apparent specificity, cytotoxic anti-HLA can also be found on occasion. As pointed out previously, contrary to the well-known hemolytic transfusion reaction that is most frequently caused by antibodies of patient origin destroying donor cells, febrile reactions can also result, and very frequently do, because of the transfusion of donor plasma containing antibodies into an unimmunized patient. Furthermore, intradonor reactions can occur in which the patient merely serves as an "incubator" for the antigen-antibody reaction. Since these febrile reactions can be severe and result in major complications, these antibodies have considerable clinical significance.

Sera that cause interference in cross-matches without contributing to red cell destruction in vivo are grouped under a blanket classification referred to as high titer, low avidity antibody (HTLA). This designation takes its name from the two outstanding features characteristically displayed by this type of serum. Sera containing such antibodies produce an equivocal type of agglutination that often defies description. Even well-trained technologists have difficulty in deciding whether or not the condition being observed is true agglutination. Reactions suspected as being positive are often described as plus-minus or even in some perhaps less scientific but nevertheless descriptive terms, such as "friendly" cells.

The second feature of such sera is the high titer. Often, antibody activity will be observed in dilutions of 1:64, 1:128, or greater. However, in contrast to the results obtained in the titration of familiar red cell antibodies in which the reactions are quite strong in the low dilutions and gradually taper off to the end point, these sera give the same degree of weak and questionable agglutination throughout the course of the dilution series. A third but less common characteristic is that if the tests are repeated using either an older test cell panel or if the test cells are prepared from a repeat specimen of blood collected from the same individual on the same day, the phenomenon disappears and the serum no longer appears to contain antibodies.

On occasion it is tempting to believe that every serum containing a so-called low avidity, high titer antibody contains antibodies to white cells. Caution is urged very strongly against accepting such an assumption as a final conclusion. A white cell antibody is, after all, a very specific entity and the fact that a serum gives peculiar reactions with red cells is no real proof that it contains white cell antibodies. Before a final conclusion is reached, sera of this type must be tested for their reactivity with white cells. Nevertheless, from a practical point of view, it is safest to transfuse such patients with packed red cells rather than with whole blood.

Before it became apparent that some of the antibodies displaying this type of behavior were in fact directed against leukocyte antigens, they were assigned to several new blood group systems, the most notable of which are Bg and Chido. Historically, the first antibody of the Bg family was anti-Donna. The serum was considered peculiar in that it reacted not only with red cells but with agglutinated white cells as well. Eventually additional sera were discovered whose antibodies all gave somewhat unusual reactions with red cells. Since this group of antibodies defied description in classical blood group terms by not defining a genetic system, they were lumped into a category called Donna-Bennet-Goodspeed or Bg.

As investigation progressed enough confidence was gained to describe three groups of antibodies in the Bg system. These were named anti-Bg^a, anti-Bg^b, and anti-Bg^c, according to the custom of blood group workers. Even though numerous examples of each of these were found, many problems persisted.

In the meantime, it became obvious that the reactions of the antibodies of the Bg system with red cells corresponded to the occurrence of certain well-known HLA antigens on the lymphocytes of the red cell donors.[14] In other studies it could be shown that under special conditions anti-Bg^a sera reacted with HLA-B7 on lymphocytes, anti-Bg^b with HLA-B17, and anti-Bg^c with HLA-A28. Naturally, the question arose as to whether the HLA antigens are already on red cells or whether the anti-Bg sera containing antibodies contain additional antibodies that react with certain specific HLA antigens. When it could be shown by absorption studies that the sera did not contain two separate antibodies the idea of some form of cross-reactivity or HLA antigen expression on red cells was explored.

Present-day evidence indicates that the antigen known as Bg^a on the red cells is in effect the HLA-B7 antigen of white cells and that they are one and the same antigen. The antigen Bg^b on the red cells is identical to the white cell antigen HLA-B17, while Bg^c is the same as the antigen known as HLA-A28. However, the HLA antigens in question are not normally present on the membrane of mature red cells, but are adsorbed from the plasma. During the normal metabolism of leukocytes, the antigens of the HLA system (especially B7, B17, and A28, for some as yet unknown reason) are shed from the cell surface and appear in the plasma as soluble antigens. These soluble antigens are found in association with the plasma lipoproteins and readily adhere to red cell surfaces. When such "coated" red cells are tested with an anti-Bg^a serum, the red cells will agglutinate, but not as firmly as would be expected in low dilutions of serum, probably because high antibody levels can strip away some of the adsorbed antigen from the cell surface. This is one of the major reasons why sera of this type give the impression of being of high titer but low avidity. They are in fact quite avid, having a high binding affinity for their antigen. It just happens that their antigen is not part of the red cell membrane.

Mechanically, the Bg antigens operate in the same fashion as the soluble Lewis antigens. By extensive washing one can make Bg positive cells Bg negative. Similarly, cells from an individual who is definitely Bg negative can be rendered Bg positive by incubating them in plasma containing the Bg antigen.

Since the quantity of soluble HLA antigen in plasma varies considerably from one day to the next, the red cells have variable amounts of this substance affixed to their surface at any given point in time. This fact goes a long way toward explaining some of the peculiarly variable reaction patterns of anti-Bg^a. If, for example, a person is being tested on a day when his or her plasma level of HLA-B7 soluble antigen is very high, his or her cells would be heavily coated with the antigen and give strong reactions. On the other hand, if the person was tested on another day when the amount of soluble antigen was very low or even absent, his or her red cells would be poorly coated and give essentially negative reactions.

Other antigens that pose similar problems are Chido (Ch^a) and Rogers (Rg^a). Like Bg, they were originally thought to be red cell membrane antigens. Shortly thereafter, they were believed to be in some way related to white cell antigens since they appeared to be genetically associated with HLA. Present-day evidence indicates that they are neither of these. Chido and Rogers are now known to be genetically controlled antigenic subclasses of the electrophoretic variants of one of the complement components, C4.[15] Chido is the slow-migrating variant C4S and Rogers is the fast-moving variant C4F. Therefore, the Chido and Rogers antigens are in effect soluble antigens. Since red cells normally possess a receptor for C4b, these antigens attach to erythrocytes and behave like true blood group antigens. In addition, since this polymorphism of C4, i.e., C4F and C4S, is controlled by alleles within the MHC, Ch^a and Rg^a show a genetic association with HLA.

Sera from patients polytransfused with whole blood or components, multiparous women, or patients who have received organ transplants may contain an anti-HLA, anticomplement, or other antibodies that upon cross-matching with the red cells of a potential donor carrying the appropriate antigens may display some unusual agglutination characteristics. When this occurs two steps must be taken. First, positive proof must be obtained that the antigen in question is not a red cell antigen. This can be done by repeating the tests, using fresh samples and extensively washed red cells. Sometimes the serum may have to be absorbed with pooled platelets, which will remove antibodies to HLA without disturbing those reactive with red cell antigens. Second, specific tests for the true identity of the offending antibody should be obtained. In any event it is safest to administer the blood as packed, washed red cells.

Review Questions

1. Describe the serological test used to detect lymphocyte antigens.
2. How is the HLA system inherited?
3. What is the difference between class I and class II MHC antigens?
4. What is the tissue distribution of the HLA-DR antigens?
5. Which HLA antigens are important in platelet transfusion?
6. What are CREGS?
7. What does the MLC test measure?
8. How are the Bg antigens related to HLA?
9. List five known neutrophile antigens.
10. Describe two pathologic conditions caused by antigranulocyte antibodies.
11. Describe the clinical significance of the P1^{A1} antigen.

REFERENCES

1. Zmijewski CM: HLA Typing in Transfusion Therapy. In Sherwood WC and Cohen A (eds): The Fetus, Infant and Child. New York, Masson, 1980.
2. Dausset J and Svejgaard A: HLA and Disease. Copenhagen, Munksgaard, 1977.
3. Amos DB and Kostyu DD: HLA—A central immunological agency of man. In Harris H and Hirschhorn K (eds): Advances in Human Genetics, Vol. 10. New York, Plenum, 1980, p 137.
4. Benacerraf B and McDevitt HO: The histocompatibility-linked immune response genes. Science 175:273, 1972.
5. Terasaki PI (ed): Histocompatibility Testing 1980. Los Angeles, UCLA Tissue Typing Laboratory, 1980.

6. Mittal KK, Mickey MR, Singal DP, and Terasaki PI: Serotyping for homotransplantation. XVIII. Refinement of microdroplet lymphocyte cytotoxicity test. Transplantation 6:913, 1968.

7. Johnson AH, Rossen RD, and Butler WT: Detection of alloantibodies using a sensitive antiglobulin microcytotoxicity test: identification of low levels of antibodies in accelerated allograft rejection. Tissue Antigens 2:215, 1972.

8. Cross DE, Whittier FC, Greiner RF, et al: Preparation of monospecific HLA antibodies from cross-reactive multispecific antisera. Tissue Antigens 8:101, 1976.

9. Duquesnoy RJ, Filip DJ, Rodey GE, et al: Successful transfusion of platelets "mismatched" for HLA antigens to alloimmunized thrombocytopenia patient. Am J Hematol 2:219, 1977.

10. Lalezari P, Nussbaum H, Gelman S, and Spaet TH: Neonatal neutropenia due to maternal isoimmunization. Blood 15:236, 1960.

11. Andrews AT, Zmijewski CM, Bowman HS, and Reihart J: Transfusion reaction with pulmonary infiltration associated with HL-A specific leukocyte antibodies. Am J Clin Pathol 66:483, 1976.

12. Shulman NR, Marder VJ, Hiller MC, and Collier EM: Platelet and leukocyte isoantigens and their antibodies: serologic, physiologic, and clinical studies. Prog Hematol 4:222, 1964.

13. Yankee RA, Grumet FC, and Rogentine GN: Platelet transfusion therapy. Selection of compatible donors by HLA. N Engl J Med 281:1208, 1969.

14. Morton JA, Pickles MM, and Sutton L: The correlation of the Bg^a blood group with the HL-A7 leukocyte group: demonstration of antigenic sites on red cells and leukocytes. Vox Sang 17:536, 1969.

15. O'Neill GH, Yank SY, Tegoli J, Berger R, and Dupont B: Chido and Rodgers blood groups are distinct components of human complement C4. Nature 273:668, 1978.

16. Baur MP and Danilovs JA: Population analysis of HLA-A, B, C, DR, and other genetic markers. In Terasaki PI (ed): Histocompatibility Testing 1980. Los Angeles, UCLA Tissue Typing Laboratory, 1980, p. 995.

17. Lalezari P and Radel E: Neutrophil-specific antigens: immunology and clinical significance. Semin Hematol 11:281, 1974.

18. van Rood JJ, van Leeuwen A, Bruning JW, and Eernisse JG: Current status of human leukocyte groups. Ann NY Acad Sci 129:446, 1966.

19. Verheugt FWA, vd Borne AEG Kr, V. Noord-Bokhorst JC, Nijenhuis LE, and Engelfriet CP: ND: A new neutrophil granulocyte antigen. Vox Sang 35:13, 1978.

20. Claass FHJ, Langerak J, Sabbe LJM, and van Rood JJ: NE1: A new neutrophil specific antigen. Tissue Antigens 13:129, 1979.

21. Thompson JS, Overlin VL, Herbick JM, Severaon CD, Claas FHJ, D'Amaro J, Burns CP, Strauss RG, and Koepke JA: New granulocyte antigens demonstrated by microgranulocytotoxicity assay. J Clin Invest 65:1431, 1980.

CHAPTER 8

Quality Control

Objectives

The goals of this chapter are to acquaint the student with:
1. The general principles of quality control in the blood bank laboratory.
2. The importance of regulatory agencies in establishing quality control minima.
3. The specific elements related to equipment, reagents, products, and personnel.

The concept of quality control is an essential component of every clinical laboratory operation. The blood bank is no exception, and because of the nature of its service, meaningful quality control measures are a prerequisite to safe operation.

When this concept was introduced initially, many laboratories instituted involved and extensive quality control measures that were time consuming, expensive, and to some extent meaningless. Often technologists were hired whose sole function was to perform quality control procedures and perform tests on previously analyzed samples submitted to the laboratory for the purpose of testing its ability to perform certain diagnostic procedures. Such practices were in part a reaction to the growing control of laboratory practices by various federal, state, and professional regulatory agencies. For example, today many blood banks in the United States located in hospitals operate under regulations set forth by the FDA (Food and Drug Administration—principle federal regulatory control), the HCFA (Health Care Finance Administration—medicine), the CLIA '67 (Clinical Laboratory Improvement Act of 1967—for interstate commerce), the state department of health (local regulatory agency), the JCAH (Joint Commission on the Accreditation of Hospitals—professional accreditation), the CAP (College of American Pathologists—professional accreditation, laboratory level), and the AABB (American Association of Blood Banks—blood bank level).

The regulations published and enforced by each of these agencies are basically the same, and every laboratory employing well-trained personnel who are dedicated to the highest principles of patient care and who follow the rules of good judgment based on knowledge and common sense should have no difficulty in complying. One key factor common to all of these regulations is quality control.

Quality control can be defined as a structured comprehensive program designed to constantly assure all parties, including the pathologist, the technologist, the physician, and the patient, that each element in a particular laboratory test is functioning exactly within the specifications of the task being performed. The elements in any given task include the equipment, the reagents, the product, and the personnel.

Since personnel collectively form an essential element in any task performed in a laboratory, it is easy to see why the idea of assigning one individual to perform quality control is not in keeping with the overall purpose of the process. Rather, a constant awareness of quality control should be an essential function of every technologist in a laboratory.

Implicit in the idea of quality control is the notion of approriate documentation and review. A permanent record of all control tests and observations is essential for several reasons. First, frequently a laboratory result may not be questioned until several months or even years after it has been reported. The permanent quality control record can be consulted in such instances to show that the reagents and equipment did function properly on the day of the test, or if they did not, the record should describe the measures that were taken to rectify the conditions. Second, if the laboratory employs several people, needless duplication of control procedures could occur unless appropriate documentation is maintained. Finally, documentation and its periodic review with an indication of corrective action is required by regulatory agencies who may regard this as a measure of laboratory performance. It is usually inferred that laboratories fastidious in their control procedures perform as well or even better in their routine work.

EQUIPMENT

Every piece of equipment used in the blood bank should be tested periodically to determine whether its performance is within specified limits. This includes all incubators, thermometers, alarms, automatic dispensing pipettes, refrigerators, freezers, centrifuges, view boxes, and microscopes. Although rarely, if ever, mentioned, room temperature requires quality control as well, since many tests are incubated or at least performed at room temperature. It is appropriate therefore to consider it as an element of equipment.

REAGENTS

Most reagents used in the blood bank, including all sera used for blood grouping and containers used for blood collection, are purchased as commercial products from a manufacturer. As such they are licensed by the Bureau of Biologics of the federal government. This licensure guarantees to the purchaser that the reagents have been manufactured according to good manufacturing practices and that the finished product meets certain minimum standards of specificity and potency that have been established for that product by regulation. To control compliance with these regulations, each manufactured lot of biologic products is tested and checked by the bureau itself. Therefore, quality control procedures designed to determine whether a fresh bottle of a reagent contains the material specified on the label is redundant. However, tests need to be done to establish that the reagent complies with the standards set forth by the laboratory itself. Further, a good quality control program will assure the users that the reagent retains its original specifications of specificity and potency throughout the useful life of any given bottle.

PRODUCTS

In contrast to other clinical laboratories, the full service blood bank is engaged in the manufacture of biologic products that are used for therapeutic purposes in humans. These include whole blood, packed red cells, frozen blood, and blood components ranging from fresh frozen plasma to platelets and white blood cells.

The manufacture of these products is regulated by the FDA and the products themselves must be licensed for shipment across state lines with the intent of sale, barter, or exchange. In addition, the blood bank profession has established certain medical criteria to be followed in making these products and has stipulated conditions for their acceptable composition. Thus each of these products in its finished form has certain standards of potency, efficacy, and safety. Consequently, stringent quality control measures must be established and followed to ensure that these products are in compliance with the established standards.

PERSONNEL

Quality control of personnel in a laboratory setting is a subject that is often either ignored or treated with calculated indifference. This attitude stems from the natural tendency of all people to resent any questions about their competence or proficiency. Still, in a setting such as the blood bank, where so much depends on the direct participation and individual judgment of the personnel involved, quality control cannot be totally ignored. From the very outset, technologists working in laboratories such as the blood bank should assume the attitude that their performance will come under close scrutiny. This should not be considered a reflection on their personal competence or scientific judgment and honesty. It just happens that repetitive tasks performed over a long period of time tend to become a matter of rote. Personnel quality control procedures can be considered as methods designed to prevent the technical staff from becoming automatons.

This may be accomplished by including regularly scheduled periodic checking of other people's work as well as the work-up of unknowns as a portion of the daily routine. In addition, participation in various proficiency testing programs should not be routinely delegated to one person in the laboratory; rather the responsibility should be rotated throughout the lab. During the course of these events, to achieve maximum benefit from the program, deficiencies should be pointed out, discussed, and corrected. To remain proficient and abreast of the state of the art, it is essential that all staff members participate in continuing education programs, ranging from workshops and seminars to the regular reading of scientific journals. Since participation in such events as lectures and seminars is considered a quality control and should be documented, it is a good idea for technologists to establish a log book for this purpose very early on in their career.

Specific procedures to be used for performing the quality control checks indicated in this chapter may be found in the reference cited. They have not been presented in detail here for a number of reasons, the primary one being that such procedures must be specifically tailored to each laboratory's needs and to some extent are subject to the individual director's professional judgment. Therefore, they will tend to vary somewhat from one laboratory to the next. However, they should be clearly defined in each institution's standard operating procedures manual. Every medical technologist should become well-versed in these methods, since, as we have attempted to indicate throughout this section, quality control is an essential aspect of every medical technologist's job.

Review Questions

1. Define quality control.
2. What is the purpose of quality control?
3. How are quality control minima established?
4. What is the key to all quality control procedures?
5. List the four elements in any given task that must be controlled.
6. What is an essential element of a good quality control program?
7. Is it necessary to quality control room temperature in blood bank work and if so, why?
8. How should blood-grouping reagents be quality controlled in the laboratory?
9. Describe a procedure for quality control of personnel.
10. What is the place of continuing education in a quality control program?

REFERENCES

1. American Association of Blood Banks: Technical Manual. 7th ed. Washington, DC, AABB, 1977.
2. American Association of Blood Banks: Quality Control in Blood Banking, Technical Workshop. Washington, DC, AABB, 1973.
3. Huestis DW, Bove JR, and Busch S: Practical Blood Transfusion. 3rd ed. Boston, Little, Brown, 1981.

CHAPTER 9

Associated Topics

Objectives

The information presented in this chapter should teach the student to:
1. Understand the meaning of forensic serology.
2. Appreciate the limitations of the routine laboratory in the performance of specialized forensic procedures.
3. Understand the underlying principles associated with the exclusion of disputed paternity.
4. Perform basic calculations that may be used to determine the probability of paternity.
5. Interpret paternity testing data in the light of certain peculiarities of the various blood group systems.
6. Appreciate that all vertebrates have blood group antigen polymorphisms.
7. Recognize that some animal blood groups are shared with those of humans.
8. Appreciate that each animal species may have one or more blood group systems that is unique to that species.

APPLICATION OF BLOOD GROUPS
TO FORENSIC PATHOLOGY

Forensic pathology is that segment of medical and paramedical science that applies biologic facts to legal problems. This facet of medicine has been an important adjunct to the solution of bizarre crimes and the protection of the rights of individuals for over 200 years. One of the first documented cases occurred in 1678, when Sir Edmundburg Godfrey was found impaled on his sword and thought to be a suicide. However, a physician, after examining the body, found the victim's neck broken and deduced that the sword thrust occurred after death. As a result, three men were incriminated, declared guilty, and hanged.

In the ensuing years, medical evidence in the form of gross pathologic findings and clever deductions based on anatomic observations coupled with sound physiologic principles began to be accepted by the courts. As a result, this science grew in importance in various kinds of criminal investigations.

A new dimension was added to this field with the discovery of immunology and the exquisite specificity of serologic reactions. Early on it was recognized that due to the relative biochemical stability and unique structure of various potentially antigenic substances, serologic methods could be used to distinguish human from animal blood stains. Pioneering investigators such as Uhlenhuth, Wasserman, and others used the ring or interface precipitation technique with antisera specific for certain corresponding proteins to identify the source of such stains. Unfortunately, cross-reactivity and poor reproducibility precluded the use of this technique as a single definitive test. In more recent years the antiglobulin inhibition test has been included as an additional, confirmatory method. In this test an antihuman serum is neutralized by serum or blood stain extracts and is then tested for its ability to agglutinate erythrocytes sensitized with incomplete antibodies. The specificity and sensitivity of this test system are somewhat better but they depend on the care with which the antiglobulin serum is prepared, and, more importantly, the species of origin of the stains being identified. This is based on the fact that proteins originating from species that are phylogenetically distant carry enough biochemically distinct features to make them easily recognized as nonhuman. However, serum proteins from phylogenetically related species such as apes or monkeys share a sufficient number of antigenic determinants to make them cross-reactive.

With the availability of microbiochemical methods for the detection of specific red cell isoenzymes and the identification of specific serum proteins, the armamentarium of the forensic scientist has been expanded. The Esterase D-isoenzymes (EsD) are an example of an enzyme system that can be used for identification. The enzyme is stable for up to six weeks in samples stored at 3C and in dried blood stains for up to four weeks. Polymorphorisms can be detected by modified thin layer electrophoresis.

Other informative red cell isoenzyme systems include phosphoglucomutase-1 (PGM_1), erythrocytic acid phosphatase (EAP), and lactate dehydrogenase (LDH), although the latter is not recommended for the identification of stains.

Typically, the modern examination of stains includes both a chemical and a serologic examination to attempt to identify the nature of the stain, its species of origin, and, if human, the individual involved.

The only legally acceptable method of identifying species is by immunologic methods. Each species is characterized by certain well-defined patterns of serum protein antigens, and specific antisera are available for their identification. Although some cross-reactivity exists, as noted previously, diffusion techniques in agar gels can be used to help in their resolution. With respect to blood stains, it is possible to distinguish menstrual blood from peripheral blood by the distribution of the LDH enzymes. Blood from fetuses can be identified by the presence of fetal hemoglobin and the race can often be deduced from the presence of abnormal hemoglobins. In addition, the blood groups can be ascertained even in dried blood stains by absorption and inhibition methods.

In this procedure, anti-A and anti-B sera of known antibody concentration are added to an unknown stain extract along with appropriate controls (e.g., extracts from unstained bits of material). After appropriate incubation, the remaining antibody level is measured and compared with the control. If concentration is lower after exposure to the stain it can be concluded that this is due to the presence of the specific antigen (A, B, or both) in the extract that neutralized the antibody in question.

Another approach is to attempt to adsorb the blood group antibodies onto the stain, prepare an eluate, and then identify the recovered antibody.

A third approach consists of the mixed agglutination technique. This method is applicable not only to stains but to other materials that either contain blood group substances or have been exposed to fluids containing blood group substances. These include fibers teased from various fabrics, hair, bits of skin or tissues, and other objects. In this test, appropriate blood-grouping antisera are allowed to incubate with the materials being examined. They are then washed and Rh_o-positive red cells that have been coated with incomplete anti-D antibody and a subagglutinating dose of antihuman globulin serum are added, incubated, and finally washed away. If the primary blood group antibody was fixed by the material being tested, the sensitized red cells will adhere, forming a *mixed agglutinate*. If, on the other hand, the primary antibody was not fixed, the antihuman globulin attached to the red cells will have nothing to bind and the cells will not adhere.

Using methods such as these, one can ascertain the ABO blood groups of stains that are very old: many of the ancient Egyptian mummies have been blood grouped. In addition, as part of the U.S. bicentennial celebration, a colleague of ours, Dr. Mitsuo Yokoyamma, using a sample of hair, was able to determine that George Washington was blood group B. This can be accomplished in large measure because of the remarkable stability of the ABH polysaccharide determinants. Although not nearly as stable, even the Rh groups in blood stains up to six weeks old can be determined. The MN antigens are detectable for up to twelve weeks.

PATERNITY TESTING

The use of blood groups in forensic work is not limited to criminal investigation. As a matter of fact, such examinations are somewhat limited and are performed in specialized laboratories of medical examiners dedicated to that type of work. A more widespread use of forensic blood grouping is in the resolution of civil cases pertaining to disputed paternity. In these cases, an unwed mother of a child accuses a man of being the father. If the father denies the allegation, the genetic information provided by the determination of the blood groups of the three individuals involved is used to resolve the case.

The resolution is based on a very simple and logical genetic premise that states that cell membrane alloantigens, isoenzymes, and heritable serum protein allotypes cannot appear in the blood of a child unless they are present in the blood of either or both of the parents. Applying this premise to a case of disputed paternity, one can say that if the putative father does not have an antigen that the child does have, which the child could not have inherited from the mother, he is excluded from consideration as the true father of that child. This is considered a first order exclusion and is positive evidence that the accused man is not the father.

If, on the other hand, the accused man does have the required antigen, he cannot be excluded. This does not prove that he is the father. It only shows that he cannot be excluded from consideration.

As knowledge progressed, a large number of genetically controlled polymorphisms in humans were discovered that could be potentially useful in handling litigation of this type. Consequently, in 1971, the American Bar Association and the American Medical Association formed a joint committee to study the implications of scientific advances in blood-typing tests and to make appropriate recommendations for their use in the determination of nonpaternity.

The 1976 report of the joint committee recommended sixty-three acceptable serologic and biochemical tests that could be used for paternity proceedings involving Caucasians, blacks, and Orientals. It recognized the admissibility of not only the serologic evidence of the probability of exclusion of paternity but also the estimate of the probability of the likelihood of paternity. It urged the adoption of standard procedures for the identification of the involved parties, the collection and identification of the blood specimens, and an acceptable serologic control program by the laboratory engaged in paternity testing.

The serologic and biochemical tests were selected to definitely establish nonpaternity in 98 of 100 men who were falsely accused. At the same time they could provide an estimate of the probability of true paternity in 99 of 100 accused men who were true fathers.

Since the use of all of the test systems was not practical because of the scarcity of the rarer antisera and the lack of biochemical expertise by the majority of the paternity testing laboratories, the committee recommended the routine use of seven blood group systems: ABO, RhHr, MNSs, Kell, Duffy, Kidd, and HLA. Their selection is based on four considerations: 1. the manufactured antisera for the six red blood cell systems are readily available and reliable; 2. the cumulative probability of exclusion is 63–72% when the six red cell systems are used (Table 1); 3. the inclusion of the HLA system because of its polymorphism increased the probability of exclusion to 91–93%; and 4. there is a reasonable probability of obtaining an exclusion in relation to the cost of the tests.

Since paternity tests involve litigation proceedings, certain extraordinary measures must be exercised in the laboratory to ensure the validity of all aspects of the final results.

TABLE 1. PERCENT CUMULATIVE PROBABILITY OF EXCLUSION FOR THE SEVEN RECOMMENDED BLOOD GROUP SYSTEMS

Antigen System	Probability of Exclusion* PE	100-PE	CPE%
ABO	.1342	86.58	13.42
MNSs	.3095	69.05	40.22
Rh	.2746	72.54	56.63
Kell	.0354	96.46	58.17
Kidd	.1869	81.31	65.99
Duffy	.1844	81.56	72.26
HLA	.78–.80[+]	22–20	93.9–94.45

* *Derived from the gene frequencies in the population.*
† *At present this value is close to 0.90 because of the large number of newly described alleles. This makes the HLA system one of the most powerful single tests for establishing nonpaternity.*

Acceptance of a Paternity Case

Paternity testing should be done only in response to a specific court order, directing the participants to appear at the laboratory for the purpose of having the blood test done. Testing can be performed when requested in writing by the participants' attorneys in concert, but should not be undertaken when the tests are requested by an attorney representing only one of the parties.

Identification Procedures for Paternity Testing

The positive identification of the individuals and of the blood samples drawn from these individuals are of the utmost importance to ensure the acceptance of the submitted laboratory reports by the courts and the attorneys. Therefore a procedure manual should be developed by the laboratory that describes the laboratory rules for accepting a paternity case, the procedures to be used to identify the individuals, including photographs, fingerprints, and footprints in the case of young infants, and the blood specimens, and the serologic tests to be done. In addition, it should describe the internal recall mechanism (audit trail) to be used to trace the events in each case from the initial identification of the individuals through the serologic testing to the actual determination of nonpaternity (exclusion) or calculation of the probability of paternity.

General Serologic Considerations

Good policy dictates that antisera from at least two manufacturers should be used for performing the blood group determination. They should be subjected to rigid quality control procedures designed to demonstrate their claimed specificity before general use and at the time of each test. Only a single participant should be tested at a time and a direct antiglobulin test should be done before the red cell typings are performed, since a positive test will nullify any red cell typings that depend on the antiglobulin procedure. When any of the participants have recently been the recipients of a transfusion of whole blood or packed red cells, the typings should be deferred until the donor red cells have been eliminated from the circulation. Finally, the blood of a mother whose infant received an exchange transfusion should be tested for the offending antibodies.

In spite of these precautions, laboratory errors may occur unless extreme care is exercised to avoid: 1. improper or inadequate identification of the participants; 2. technical errors resulting from the use of inadequate antisera and controls, especially in those systems in which rigid standards from potency have not been established; and 3. human errors resulting from improper transcription or accidental transposition of results.

Special consideration regarding the ABO system. The ABO blood groups of the participants are determined directly in the standard manner with anti-A, anti-B, and anti-A, B antisera and confirmed using group A_1, B and O red cells. In addition, the anti-A_1 lectin (*Dolichos biflorus*) is used to distinguish A_1 from A_2 and A_1B from A_2B. The anti-H lectin (*Ulex europeous*) is used to determine the presence or absence of H antigen on group O and A_1 red blood cells when anti-H antibodies are suspected of being present in the sera of these blood types. Group O red cells that fail to react with the anti-H lectin belong to the rare O_h (Bombay) blood group. Group A_2 red cells may be used to confirm the presence of anti-A_1 antibodies in the serum of group A_2 and A_2B individuals.

When a discrepancy is encountered between the direct red cell typing and the indirect plasma (confirmation) typing, particularly when the group O reagent red cells react with the individual's plasma, the presence of auto- and/or alloantibodies should be considered. Their presence and specificity should be confirmed before the results of the primary direct and indirect typings are interpreted.

In addition, the existence of primary agammaglobulinemia or acquired hypogammaglobulinemia should be suspected if the appropriate anti-A and/or anti-B antibodies are undetectable. A serum protein electrophoresis and the quantitation of the immunoglobulins can serve as an aid to resolve this problem.

Occasionally, direct ABO red cell testing discrepancies may be encountered because of some disease processes. For example, antigens may be "lost" in certain leukemias or acquired in gastrointestinal malignancies or infections with E. coli.

Several important points should be considered when determining the subgroups of A. Because the A antigens are not fully developed in children less than one year old, they may give the erroneous impression of being A_2. Since Orientals are rarely group A_2, subgrouping is not a routine procedure, unless the paternity case involves an interracial couple. There appears to be an excess of groups A_2 and A_2B in the black population. This apparent excess could be due to a weak expression of the H gene resulting in a deficiency of substrate for A_1 gene-controlled enzymes. This effect is even more pronounced in AB individuals. The result is a reduced number of A_1 antigenic receptor sites on the cell surface, which leads to false negative reactions with anti-A_1 reagents. Therefore, the definition of the subgroups of A in black people is unreliable and should not be used as a basis for exclusion.

Special considerations regarding the Rh system. Six commercially available antisera generally are used to determine the Rh phenotype. These include anti-D (Rh$_o$), anti-C (rh'), and anti-E (rh''), and anti-c (hr'), anti-e (hr''), and anti-C^w (rh^w). The testing scheme may be expanded with the use of anti-f (hr), which will distinguish CDe/cDe (R^{1}R^2) from CDE/cde (R^{z}r) and Cde/cdE (r'r'') from CdE/cde (r^{y}r). However, this antiserum, which reacts with cells only when c and e are in coupling, is not generally available.

The determination of probable Rh genotypes is usually clear when the rules described in an earlier chapter are followed. Some caution should be exercised in this respect among Chinese because of the high incidence of Rh gene deletions peculiar to them. The presence of such dilutions may lead to false conclusions of not only nonpaternity but also of nonmaternity. When Chinese nonpaternity or nonmaternity is suspected, it is necessary to perform antiserum titrations in an effort to ascertain gene dosage effects before definitive conclusions can be reached.

Special considerations regarding the MNSs group. The MNSs phenotypes can be identified through readily available anti-M, anti-N, anti-S, and anti-s sera. Usually the specific genotypic combinations can be deduced from the antigens in the mother and the child. Even if this is not possible, however, the antigens can be used separately to determine the paternal obligatory gene.

Special precautions should be taken in interpreting the results in blacks because of the relatively frequent incidence of the S^u allele. This allele behaves like an amorph and fails to result in the production of either S or s antigens. Consequently, the possibility must be considered that blacks who type only with anti-S or anti-s are either SS^u or sS^u rather than SS or ss, respectively. Some workers advocate the use of an anti-U serum to prove the absence of S and s antigens since this antibody reacts with all cells that have either of them. However, since S- and s-negative individuals have been reported who react with anti-U, some question is raised about the usefulness of this reagent.

There are additional alleles of M and N that must be taken into consideration when reporting the MN phenotypes and genotypes. Two in particular are M^g and M^k, since individuals with these alleles fail to react with normal anti-M antisera. The M^g allele gives rise to a special M^g antigen, for which antisera are available. To date it has been demonstrated exclusively in Swiss families. The M^k allele is thought to be either an amorphic gene or the result of a defect in the system. The presence of M^k inhibits the production of both the MN and the Ss antigens.

Special considerations regarding the Kell system. The two antisera anti-K and anti-k are used in paternity testing in Caucasians. Generally they can define the three phenotypes KK, Kk, kk and the corresponding genotypes without difficulty. However, because of the antigen frequencies this system contributes little to the overall probability of exclusion in whites and even less in blacks. Since the Kell antigen is absent from the Chinese and Japanese, its ascertainment is omitted unless the paternity proceedings involve interracial cases.

Special considerations regarding the Duffy system. Anti-Fy^a and anti-Fy^b are the two antisera routinely used to define this blood group system. In whites and blacks, the two antisera define four phenotypes—Fy(a+b−), Fy(a+b+), Fy(a−b+), and Fy(a−b−)—that may result from one of the six corresponding genotypes: Fy^aFy^a, Fy^aFy, Fy^bFy^b, Fy^bFy, Fy^aFy^b $FyFy$. Although $FyFy$ is common in blacks, it is extremely rare in Caucasians. The three genotypes, Fy^aFy^a, Fy^aFy^b, and Fy^bFy^b, are commonly found in Orientals.

The existence of the amorphic gene Fy, which does not code for the production of any serologically detectable phenotypic product, as well as this gene's high frequency in blacks, poses certain problems in interpreting the genetics of this system. For example, when a black child is type Fy(a−b−), $Fy\ Fy$, with a mother who is Fy(a+b−), and the alleged father is Fy(a−b+), the interpretation is twofold. If the Fy (a−b+) phenotype of the alleged father is the result of the $Fy\ Fy^b$ genotype, he cannot be excluded. On the other hand, if it is the result of the Fy^bFy^b genotype, he is definitely excluded. This stems from the fact that the mother's genotype is Fy^aFy and the child's second Fy had to have been inherited from the father.

Problems of this type can be resolved with antiserum titrations, since the Duffy antigens show remarkable gene dose effects. The anti-Fy^a and anti-Fy^b antisera are titrated against the cells of the mother and the alleged father, and with cells of the known phenotypes Fy(a+b+), Fy(a+b−), and Fy(a−b+). If the titration score obtained with the alleged father's cells is equal to or greater than that obtained with the known Fy(a−b+) cell, he is of the genotype Fy^bFy^b. On the other hand, if it is less than this value and comparable to the score obtained with the known Fy(a+b+) cell, then in all probability he is the heterozygote Fy^bFy.

Special considerations regarding the Kidd system. Extreme care must be exercised when testing for the Kidd antigens because of the instability of the antibodies. Controls should be employed to document their activity each time the antisera are used.

Anti-Jk^a and anti-Jk^b define four phenotypes, Jk(a+b−), Jk(a+b+), Jk(a−b+), Jk(a−b−), and six genotypes: Jk^aJk^a, Jk^aJk, Jk^aJk^b, Jk^bJk^b, Jk^bJk, $JkJk$. The three genotypes Jk^aJk, Jk^bJk, and $JkJk$ are extremely rare in Caucasians, although they have been reported in the Chinese and Polynesians.

Special considerations regarding minus-minus phenotypes. The occurrence of minus-minus blood group phenotypes in a variety of systems among Orientals, Polynesians, and blacks must be considered as a possibility when apparent nonpaternity is based on the absence of appropriate antigens in the putative father.

A minus-minus phenotype may be the result of either a loss or translocation of a portion of a chromosome bearing a specific blood group gene. It may also be the result of homozygous amorphic genes, which do not code for any phenotypic characteristic. Examples of phenotypes resulting from the presence of amorphic genes include O_h(Bombay), Rh$_{null}$, S^u, Fy(a−b−), and Jk(a−b−).

Special considerations regarding HLA. HLA typing is performed on viable peripheral blood lymphocytes using antisera that for the most part must be prepared by the individual user. In addition, cross-reactivity and subtleties in HLA antigen expression that occur in various races demand expert attention in performance and interpretation. Therefore, the use of this system in paternity cases is ordinarily restricted to highly specialized centers that possess the necessary reagents and expertise.

Estimation of the Probability in Favor of Paternity

Up to this point, various procedures have been discussed that can be used to establish an exclusion, that the accused man cannot possibly be the father of the child in question because he does not have one or more genetic characteristics that the child had to have inherited from its true father. Suppose, however, that regardless of the extent of testing such an exclusion is not possible. Even in this case it is still not possible to accuse the putative father with certainty. However, it is possible to estimate the probabililty of his being the true father.

The probability can be computed in a number of different ways. One of the most widely used compares the frequency of the "obligatory genes" in the accused man, x, with the frequency of the "obligatory genes" in a population of random individuals of the same race, y. These gene frequencies correspond to probabilities. Thus the total probability corresponds to the cummulative product of the gene frequencies for each of the obligatory genes under consideration.

A sample of this type of data is shown in Table 2. The alleged father in this case cannot be excluded since he possesses all of the obligatory genes. Since he is homozygous for these genes in the ABO, Rh, Kell, and MN systems, the probability of his passing them on to his offspring is 100% or 1.0000. He is heterozygous for the appropriate gene in the remaining systems, and therefore the probability of passing on any one of these is 50% or 0.5000. The combined probability of his transmitting

TABLE 2. CASE A: CALCULATION OF THE PROBABILITY OF PATERNITY IN A CASE OF NONEXCLUSION

Mother	Child	Paternal Obligatory Genes (O.G.)	Alleged Father (A.F.)	Freq. O.G.'s A.G.	Freq. O.G.'s Random Man
B	0	0	0	1.0000	0.6604
DCc̄ee	ddc̄c̄ee	dc̄e	ddc̄c̄ee	1.0000	0.3998
kk	kk	k	kk	1.0000	0.9640
MMSS	MMSS	MS,Mu	MMSS	1.0000	0.2584
Fy(a+b+)	Fy(a−b+)	Fy^b,Fy	Fy(a+b+)	0.5000	0.4251
Jk(a+b−)	Jk(a+b+)	Jk^b	Jk(a+b+)	0.5000	0.4899
HLA-A-2,3	A-2,11	A-11	A-1,11	0.5000	0.0619
HLA-B-5,15	B-15,18	A-18	B-7,18	0.5000	0.0513

$$x = 0.0625 \quad y = 0.000004945$$

$$W = \frac{x}{x + y} = \frac{.0625}{.0625 + .000004945} \times 100 = 99.99\%$$

$$PI = 12{,}639$$

N.B. In legal work, the antigen c̄ is annotated with a bar so as to distinguish it from C.

TABLE 3. CALCULATION OF THE PROBABILITY OF PATERNITY IN A CASE OF EXCLUSION BASED ON HLA

Mother	Child	O.G.	A.F.	O.G.(A.F.)	O.G.(R.M.)
B	B	B,O	A_2B	0.5000	0.8254
Dc̄c̄ee	Dc̄c̄ee	Dc̄e,dc̄e	Dc̄c̄ee	1.0000	0.7241
kk	kk	k	kk	1.0000	0.9962
MNs̄s̄	MNS^{u}S^u	MS^u, MS^u	MNS^{u}S^u	1.0000	0.1237
Fy(a−b+)	Fy(a−b+)	Fy^b,Fy	Fy(a−b−)	1.0000	0.9191
Jk(a+b+)	Jk(a+b+)	JK^a,Jk^b	JK(a+b−)	1.0000	1.0000
A-30,31	A-3,30	A-3	A-1,28		
				EXCLUSION	
B-17,42	B-1,17	B-7	B-x,x		
				0.5000	0.06769
				W = 88.07%	
				PI = 7.39	

all of the obligatory genes is .1 × .1 × .1 × .1 × .5 × .5 × .5 × .5 or 0.0625. This is equal to x. The figures in the random man column are the gene frequencies of the obligatory genes in the population, and the product is equal to y. The chances of the accused man being the true father can be expressed as either the plausibility of paternity (W) or the paternity index (PI). In this case the values are quite high— 99.99% and 12,639 respectively. Nevertheless, it must be understood that in spite of this result, definite proof of paternity has not been obtained. Therefore these values are not acceptable as evidence in favor of paternity by most courts. However, they are frequently helpful in bringing about an out-of-court settlement.

The magnitude and ranges of these values can be appreciated from the data obained in case B shown in Table 3. In this case, the alleged father is excluded on the basis of the HLA system. Nevertheless, if this system had not been considered, the W equals 88.07% and the PI equals 7.39, values that are almost borderline in favor of paternity.

ANIMAL BLOOD GROUPS

Alloantigens of erythrocytes capable of classifying individuals into various groups are not confined to humans but are found among all members of the animal kingdom. As in humans, these characteristics are of considerable importance when it becomes necessary to perform a blood transfusion. Transfusion in veterinary practice is not all that uncommon, especially in large medical centers, and may arise in two vastly different situations. In some cases, a pet may develop an anemia due to illness or require some form of surgery that could necessitate a therapeutic blood transfusion. In other cases, and these are the most frequent episodes, animals used for experimental purposes in whom an investigator has invested considerable time and money may suffer sudden and unexpected blood loss as the result of manipulative procedures. Sophisticated veterinary hospitals are not always accessible in a vivarium and the frustrated investigator, usually a surgeon, will turn to his friends in the blood bank for aid.

Apart from these unusual emergency circumstances, the blood groups of animals are interesting in their own right. Any serious student of blood-grouping science can benefit from even a superficial knowledge of their expression and methods of detection.

The subject of animal blood groups can be conveniently partitioned into three categories: 1. blood groups associated with all members of the animal kingdom; 2. blood groups in lower animals shared with those of humans; and 3. red cell polymorphism unique to a given species.

Interspecies Antigens

The typical example of a polymorphism expressed on the red cells of all animals is the Forssman antigen, originally discovered in 1911.[1] This antigen is better classified as a tissue antigen rather than a blood group antigen, since it is found in the tissues of the solid organs as well as on the red cells. Therefore, from that standpoint the Forssman system occupies a position identical with that of the ABO system in humans.

The entire animal kingdom can be divided into Forssman "positive" or Forssman "negative," depending on the occurrence of the antigen in the tissues (Table 4). Two animals, the guinea pig and the sheep, are unique. The guinea pig, although Forssman positive, has no Forssman antigen on its red cells. The sheep, on the other hand, is classified as Forssman negative since it has no antigen in its tissues. However, it does express the Forssman antigen on its red cells.

The Forssman antigen apparently exhibits some structural relationship to the cell-bound ABH antigens of humans and is ubiquitous in nature. For this reason most Forssman negative animals have anti-Forssman antibodies in their sera. These are complement-binding antibodies and can cause hemolytic transfusion reactions if intraspecies blood replacement is attempted without regard to this barrier. This antigen does have some significance in the clinical laboratory setting. During the course of infectious mononucleosis, a disease of humans, antibodies are developed that agglutinate sheep red blood cells. These are often referred to as heterophile an-

TABLE 4. DISTRIBUTION OF THE FORSSMAN ANTIGEN

Positive Species	Negative Species
Guinea Pig*	Rabbit
Horse	Human
Dog	Ox
Cat	Rat
Mouse	Fowl (Goose, Pigeon)
Fowl (Chicken)	Eel
Tortoise	Frog
	Sheep**

  * Positive animal but lacks antigen on red cells.
** Negative animal but expresses antigen on red cells only.

tibodies and are most likely produced as a result of cross-reactivity. The presence of such heterophile agglutinations in the patient's serum is a useful tool in establishing the diagnosis of the disease. However, because humans have anti-Forssman antibodies, their sera will react with the Forssman-bearing sheep erythrocytes. Therefore, these antibodies must be removed by absorption using a Forssman positive tissue, such as guinea pig kidney, prior to testing for the heterophile antibody of infectious mononucleosis.

Antigens Shared with Humans

The blood groups found in lower animals that are shared with those of humans are for the most part associated with the ABO blood group system. The Rh groups or antigens intimately associated with them are found in some of the higher primates as well. However, ABO is in the majority by far. As might be inferred from the known cross-reactivity, most animal species possessing A-like or B-like antigens belong to the Forssman positive group.

Hogs. Many hogs belong to blood group A. In addition to carrying this antigen on their red cells, these animals can exhibit them in their secretions. Hog gastric mucosa is a rich source of A-like antigen. The A antigen purified from this material is used to hyperimmunize human volunteers for the production of potent anti-A typing reagents.[2] In addition, it can be employed to neutralize unwanted anti-A in commercial preparations of alloantisera to other human blood group antigens, such as Rh, Kell, Duffy, etc.

  The A antigen of hogs, though related to human A antigen, appears to be slightly different. The so-called A^P antigen found on the erythrocytes of hogs reacts with the human "immune" anti-A formed as a result of alloimmunization of pregnancy, even though the purified substance from gastric mucosa fails to do so.

Horses. Some horses belong to the humanlike blood group AB, although they seem to have more B-like than A-like antigens. The gastric mucosa of this species serves as a source of antigen that when purified can be used to neutralize human anti-B antibody.

Rabbits. Rabbits are either group A-like or non-group A-like, depending on the presence of the appropriate antigen in their organs. Since A-like rabbits are also secretors it is possible to ascertain their status by means of a saliva inhibition of agglutination test. This fact could have some bearing on the use of rabbits for the production of antibodies against a variety of human antigens.

  One of the difficulties encountered in these procedures is that to be of any value rabbit antisera must first be absorbed to remove nonspecific antihuman activity. Lambert[3] pointed out many years ago that the production of such unwanted antibodies can be greatly reduced by preselecting the animals to be immunized. So, for example, non-group A-like rabbits tend to produce a large quantity of nonspecific antihuman antibodies, the majority of which are anti-A. The group A-like animals, on the other hand, tend to produce considerably less nonspecific antihuman antibodies and no anti-A at all.

Apparently unrelated to the presence of A-like antigen in the tissues, B-like antigen is carried by some rabbits on their red cells. This antigen is called B^R and is capable of absorbing naturally occurring anti-A from group B human sera.[4]

Dogs. Certain breeds of dogs secrete A-like or B-like antigens in their saliva. These antigens do not cause transfusion problems since they are not expressed on red cells. However, they may occasionally present problems in forensic work, when one is attempting to identify the blood groups of an assailant from sweat-stained cloth. If, for example, the stained cloth had been mouthed by a stray dog in the vicinity, the resultant blood group determination could be obscured or present a confusing picture due to the presence of A or B antigens from canine saliva.

Primates. As might be expected, various species of lower primates are the most frequent carriers of human A-like and B-like antigens. Among them, chimpanzees and orangutans carry classical antigens on their red cells fully reactive with normal human blood-grouping reagents, and naturally occurring antibodies in their sera.[5, 6]

Approximately 90% of chimpanzees belong to blood group A and the remaining 10% to group O. To date the B antigen has not been found among chimpanzees. In addition, chimpanzees also exhibit the D and C antigens of the Rh blood group system as well as the M antigen of the MN system. Chimpanzee red cells react with *Vicea graminea* lectin, and so are believed to have an antigen called N^V.

Orangutans, on the other hand, can be of group A, B, or AB. None tested has been found belonging to a group corresponding to O. Some members of this species also exhibit an M-like antigen. Gibbons, like orangutans, can be A, B, or AB. In addition they have both M and N but only c of the Rh system.

Other species of primates, such as gorillas, baboons, and certain types of monkeys, exhibit the ABH antigens only in their secretions. Most of these animals have the expected anti-A or anti-B in their sera. On this basis, mountain gorillas belong to blood group A whereas lowland gorillas belong to blood group B. Rhesus monkeys secrete a human B-like antigen and normally have anti-A, whereas Java monkeys are principally group A. Some group O Java monkeys have been found, as well as others that appear to be AB. Interestingly, in this case the AB antigens seem to be inherited through a single AB allele.

Species-Specific Alloantigens

The third class of animal blood groups are the species-specific alloantigens. These alloantigens, like those of humans, are capable of distinguishing among different individuals of the same species.

For the most part these antigens are expressed as *allo* antigens only in a given species. In other species these very same antigens may be found as nonpolymorphic characteristics. This leads to a very interesting concept—some membrane structures found on the red cells of every single member of one species (monomorphism) may be found on the cells of only a certain proportion of another species (polymorphism), thus displaying the properties of an allospecificity.

Usually, the antigens are detected with antisera that are the products of cross-species xenoimmunization. Occasionally, however, alloimmune sera can be used for their detection. Naturally occurring antibodies are not normally found. As with all other examples of alloantigenic polymorphisms, these characteristics are under genetic control within any given species.

Dogs. The use of dogs as experimental animals for developing new surgical procedures necessitated periodic intraspecies transfusion, which sometimes resulted in hemolytic reactions. This prompted a number of investigators to study canine blood groups by means of deliberate alloimmunization. A number of systems have been discovered, among them Aa, Bb, Cc, Dd, Ee, F, and G.[7] The A system, which bears no resemblance to human A, is the most powerful. About 60% of dogs are A-"positive," making this antigen and its antibody responsible for the majority of reactions in polytransfused animals.

Rabbits. Cohen[7] has studied rabbits extensively and has defined at least three major antigenic systems—A, D, and F—using alloimmune sera. In addition, some rabbits have a compound antigen composed of AF that is called J and another composed of AD that is called I.

Rats. Certain inbred strains of laboratory rats were originally studied by Owen and later by Palm (see ref. 7). One interesting polymorphism was found in which rats either had an antigen called A or its antibody called alpha (α), but not both. Later antigenic characteristics called C, D, E, and F were described. Since that time rat erythrocytes have been shown to carry a host of other polymorphisms. Since this species is enjoying immense popularity as an experimental animal in many biomedical laboratories, undoubtedly a host of complex genetic systems will emerge.

Mice. The predominant polymorphic characteristics carried by mouse red cells are the antigens of the H-2 system. Interestingly, the H-2 antigens are gene products of the mouse major histocompatibility complex and therefore behave as transplantation antigens. Thus, unlike humans and other species in whom the histocompatibility antigens are restricted to nucleated cells, the mouse expresses them on the red cells as well. Because of the importance of the mouse in the study of transplantation and its use as the primary experimental animal for the study of immunologic phenomena, the H-2 system is the most thoroughly explored of all animal erythrocyte polymorphisms and several major reference works have been written on the subject. The reader is encouraged to explore this fascinating system in more detail.

Sheep. Red cell antigens of sheep have been studied extensively by Rasmussen and others.[7] Even though these animals possess many alloantigens of red cells, two of them, M and L, are particularly interesting. There is a physiologic characteristic among sheep that has to do with the amount of potassium normally found in their red cells. Some of the animals, called HK, have a normally high potassium level whereas others, called LK, normally exhibit low potassium levels. Studies have revealed that HK animals are blood group L. At present it is not known whether the presence of these antigens contributes directly to the manner in which potassium passes through the cell membrane or whether the genes responsible for antigen production are linked and in disequilibrium with those controlling the potassium pump.

Cats. Cats have been studied by Holmes and by Eyquem.[7] In this species normal or naturally occurring alloantibodies occur. Use of these normal sera made it possible to define two major antigens, referred to as A or EF and B or O, depending on the author. All the cats studied were either A or B; the combination AB or the total absence of either was not found. Since naturally occurring antibodies do occur, they can be of significance in transfusion between different breeds.

Pigs. A number of pig red cell alloantigens have been described, among them A, Ka, B, Ea, Eb, C, F, EaEe, X, and Y.[7] The frequency distribution varies considerably among different species. These antigens are of considerable importance in countries such as Poland, since selective breeding has resulted in ham and other pork products being one of that nation's leading exports. Hog farmers are quite protective of their breeding stocks. Therefore, the major usefulness of the pig red cell alloantigenic markers is in the settlement of disputed paternity arising from illegal breeding.

Cattle. Cattle blood groups have been studied extensively by Stormont.[7] The major systems include A, B, C, F-V, J, L, M, N, S, Z, and R′-S′. The J system results in the formation of soluble antigens that become attached to red cells somewhat like the Lewis antigens in humans. To define the antigens of this system, antibodies from five different sera are required. As a matter of fact, the definition of most of the cattle blood groups demands the availability of a battery of sera from different sources, as shown in Table 5. Further testimony upholding the complexity of cattle alloantigens is given by the number of factors in the B system listed in Table 6.

TABLE 5. SOURCES OF SERA NORMALLY NEEDED TO DEFINE CATTLE BLOOD GROUPS

Cattle alloimmune	Rabbit anti-human A*
Rabbit anti-cattle	Cattle anti-human A*
Sheep alloimmune	Normal antelope
Normal cattle*	Sheep anti-cattle
Normal sheep*	Goat anti-cattle
Normal goat*	

* Sera required to define the J system.

TABLE 6. FACTORS IN THE B-SYSTEM OF CATTLE[7]

B_1	O_x	D'	Y'
B_2	P	E_2'	B'
G	P_2	E_3'	NF7
G_2-T_3	Q	E_x'	O'
I	T_1	F'	S_2
I_2	Y_1	G'	S5
K	Y_2	I'	S27
O_1	A_1	J'	S34
O_3	A_2	K'	
		O'	

Primates. An extensive series of primate species-specific alloantigenic polymorphisms has been described. The reader is referred to reviews by Wiener et al.[5] One of the most interesting is the V-A-B system. An antibody to one of the antigens of this system was originally produced by immunizing a chimpanzee with human red cells. Another antibody to a second antigen of this system was produced by immunizing a different chimpanzee with the red cells of the same human. Therefore, it must be concluded that the human cells carried all of the alloantigens of this system and the antibody produced depended on the alloantigenic makeup of the antibody producer.

The nature of allospecificity and the question of why a given structure is polymorphic in one species and monomorphic in another are subjects that are quite thought provoking. The result of the immunization of chimpanzees with human red cells is but one bit of evidence indicating that this situation can exist. Another example can be derived from an examination of the sources of sera used for the identification of cattle blood groups.

Three species, rabbit, sheep, and goat, each recognize a different antigenic structure on cattle red cells, so that the resultant antisera define polymorphisms in cattle. This is relatively easy to understand, but why should normal anti-antelope serum recognize polymorphisms among cattle?

In some newer work along these same lines, rats of the BN strain were immunized with cells from rats of the Lewis strain. After appropriate hybridization, monoclonal antibodies were produced and analyzed. Among the repertoire of antibodies produced as the result of this immunization were some that not only detected polymorphisms among rats, as might be expected, but also among mice and even among humans.[8]

This topic offers a great deal of material for reflection on a rainy Sunday afternoon.

Review Questions

1. What would you conclude from these family study results?

Putative father	A₁ MN	CčDEe
Mother	O N	Cčdee
Child 1	A₂ N	CčDee
Child 2	A₁ MN	ččdee

   Putative father A_1 MN CčDEe
   Mother   O N   Cčdee
   Child 1 A_2 N   CčDee
   Child 2 A_1 MN   ččdee

2. The Rh types of this family study were uninformative.

	GROUP	AGE
Putative father	A_2	30 yrs
Mother	O	25 yrs
Child	A_1	3 mos

   What is your conclusion regarding paternity?

3. For each of the following cases, state whether the accused man can or cannot be *excluded* as the father of the baby.

	BABY	MOTHER	ACCUSED MAN
1.	MN	N	MN
2.	O	B	A_1
3.	CDe/cde	cde/cde	čDE/čde
4.	A CDe/cde	A CDe/CDe	O CDe/CDe

4. What is the meaning of cumulative probability of exclusion?
5. What is the meaning of estimate of the probability of true paternity?
6. Describe the principles underlying the identification procedures used in paternity cases.
7. List two conditions that should be considered when interpreting the ABO groups in paternity tests.
8. Describe the basic principle used in estimating the likelihood of paternity.
9. What is the Forssman antigen?
10. Which known blood group antigens are also found in animals?

REFERENCES

1. Wilson GS and Miles AA: Topley and Wilson's Principles of Bacteriology and Immunity. 4th ed. London, Arnold, 1957, p 1239.
2. Witebsky E: Isolation and purification of blood group A and B substances, their use in conditioning universal donor blood, in neutralizing anti-Rh sera, and in the production of potent grouping sera. Science 46:887, 1946.

3. Lambert RM: Personal communication, 1956.
4. Yokoyama M and Stegmaier A: A new method for detection of "immune" type of anti-B antibody. Proc Soc Exp Biol Med 119:854, 1965.
5. Wiener AS, Socha WW, and Moor-Jankowski J: Homologues of the human A-B-O blood groups in apes and monkeys. Haemalotogia (Budap) 8:195, 1974.
6. Socha WW and Moor-Jankowski J: Blood groups of anthropoid apes and their relationship to human blood groups. J Human Evol 8:453, 1979.
7. Cohen C and Amos DB (eds): Blood groups in infrahuman species. Ann NY Acad Sci 97, Art. 1, pp 1–328, 1962.
8. Boyd HC, Smilek DE, Spielman RS, Zmijewski CM, and McKearn TJ: Monoclonal rat anti-MHC alloantibodies detect HLA-linked polymorphisms in humans. Immunogen 12:313, 1981.

SELECTED BIBLIOGRAPHY

American Association of Blood Banks: Paternity Testing. A seminar presented by the Committee on Technical Workshops. Washington, DC, AABB, 1978.
Gonzales A, Vance M, Helpern M, and Umberger J: Legal Medicine, Pathology and Toxicology: Examination of Blood. 2nd ed. New York, Appleton-Century-Crofts, 1954, Ch 26, p 622.
Gradwohl's Legal Medicine: Identification by Trace Evidence, Ch 12, p 154. 3rd ed. Camps FE (ed). A. John Wright and Sons Ltd. Publication. Distributed by Year Book Medical Publications, Inc., Chicago, 1976.
Knight B: Blood Identification. Vol II. Physical Trauma. Tedeschi CG, Eckert WG, and Tedeschi LG (eds): Forensic Medicine. Philadelphia, W.B. Saunders, 1977 Ch 26, p 810.
Miale JB et al (eds): Joint AMA-ABA guidelines: present status of serologic testing in problems of disputed parentage. Family Law QX:247, 1976.
Polesky HF: Paternity Testing. Chicago, ASCP-EMS, 1975.
Sussman LN: Paternity Testing. 2nd ed. Springfield, Ill, C.C. Thomas, 1976.

Selected Routine Methods

GENERAL TESTS FOR RED CELL ANTIGENS

Red cell antigens can be detected by means of commercially available red cell grouping reagents. To a large extent, the exact procedures to be employed with respect to time and temperature of incubation, cell-suspending media, and the use of the indirect antiglobulin procedure will depend on the manufacturer's specific instructions. Deviation from such directions can lead to completely erroneous results and on occasion may be illegal. Generally, such tests can be divided into either slide tests or tube tests.

Slide Tests

1. Place one drop of antiserum within the confines of a wax ring drawn on a flat, clean glass plate.
2. Add a small amount of blood (see below) to the drop of antiserum using clean applicator sticks or Pasteur pipettes. Blood specimens may be taken from the finger tip or by venipuncture and may be either clotted or in some suitable anticoagulant. When applicator sticks are used, the amount of blood transferred should produce an approximate 3% suspension in the final serum-cell mixture. Note: When using red cells from a macerated blood clot, be careful not to transfer small clots into the antisera. Although in some instances (e.g., blood from newborns) a 10% saline suspension of washed red cells may be used, saline-suspended red cells are not recommended for routine slide testing.

3. The contents of the wax rings are thoroughly mixed with clean wooden applicator sticks, and the slide is rocked gently by hand and observed macroscopically for agglutination. In some instances (testing for Rh but not ABO), a light-heated viewing box may be helpful. However, care must be exercised that the temperature on the glass plate does not exceed 45–47 C, as excessive temperature may disperse or weaken agglutination.

4. Reading should be done before drying occurs: three minutes is the maximum time. The use of glass rods for mixing slide tests should be avoided. Such a procedure can cause minute amounts of colloidal silica to be released, which can cause spontaneous clumping of cells, especially when the antisera consist of very dilute protein solutions.[1]

Tube Tests

1. Prepare a 2% suspension of once-washed cells in the appropriate diluent.
2. Add one drop of the antiserum to a small test tube (10 × 75 mm), appropriately labeled.
3. Add one drop of the 2% cell suspension and mix the contents thoroughly by gentle shaking.
4. Incubate the tubes for the required length of time at the recommended temperature, then centrifuge for thirty seconds in a small, high speed centrifuge such as a Sero-Fuge (Clay-Adams) or equivalent at 3,400 rpm.
5. After centrifugation, shake the tubes gently to dislodge the cell button. The degree of agglutination is judged macroscopically according to the number and size of the clumps and the number of free cells (Fig. 1). A magnifying mirror or a hand lens may be used to aid in reading the reactions in the tube method. Microscopic readings are generally not necessary, except when a mixed cell field (some cells agglutinated, others free) is suspected or expected. If this is to be carried out, the resuspended red cells are gently transferred with a pipette to a glass slide and examined under the low power objective of the microscope.

Care must be taken in shaking the tubes as some antisera produce very

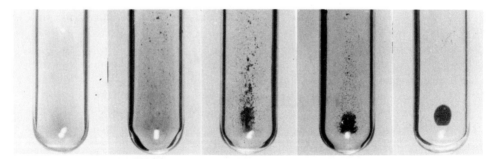

Fig. 1. Degrees of red cell agglutination as seen in test tube tests; from left to right: − (negative), +, ++, +++, ++++.

delicate agglutinates that can be readily dispersed by vigorous shaking. On the other hand, cell suspensions in viscous diluents such as bovine albumin may be difficult to dislodge. To avoid difficulties in interpretation, it is mandatory that diluent controls, consisting of one drop of cell suspension and one drop of diluent, be used in all tube tests.

ERYTHROCYTE ANTIBODY SENSITIZATION TESTS

Direct Antiglobulin Test (Test for In Vivo Sensitization of Red Cells)

1. Prepare a 2% cell suspension in saline from a clotted sample of blood.
2. Wash two drops of this suspension four times with 2.5 ml of cold saline in a 10×75 mm tube.
3. After the last wash, decant the supernatant saline as completely as possible.
4. Add two drops of antihuman globulin serum and resuspend the cell button in the serum by tapping the tube gently.
5. Centrifuge for fifteen seconds at 3,400 rpm in a Sero-Fuge (Clay-Adams) or equivalent.
6. Read macroscopically for agglutination (Fig. 1).

Indirect Antiglobulin Test (Test for In Vitro Sensitization of Red Cells)

1. Prepare a 2% cell suspension in saline from a clotted or anticoagulated sample of blood.
2. Place two drops of cell suspension in a 10×75 mm test tube.
3. Add two drops of the diagnostic antiserum (e.g., anti-K) or unknown serum to be tested for the presence of incomplete antibodies.
4. Incubate for thirty minutes at 37 C or according to the specifications supplied by the manufacturer.
5. Continue with step 2 of the direct antiglobulin test.

LOW IONIC STRENGTH—INDIRECT ANTIGLOBULIN TEST
(Modified by Moore and Mollison[2])

Reagents:

1. Low-ionic strength solution (LISS). (Conductivity 3.7 mmho/cm at 23 C, NaCl-0.03 M)
   180 ml saline 0.17 M

20 ml phosphate buffer 0.15 M, ph 6.7 (Equal volumes 0.15 M Na_2HPO_4 + 0.15 M Na_2PO_4)

800 ml glycine [36% w/v in H_2O (adjusted to pH 6.7 with 1.0 M NaOH)] Distribute the LISS into small aliquots and sterilize immediately, since nonsterile LISS stored at 4 C is an excellent medium for bacterial growth. Maintain the PBS in the refrigerator when not being used. Allow the LISS and PBS to come to room temperature before using. The pH is critical and should be checked daily.

2. Phosphate buffered saline solution (PBSS) pH 6.7.
3. 3% red blood cell concentration is LISS:
   a. Wash the red blood cells twice with phosphate buffered saline.
   b. Wash once in LISS: dilute washed red cells in LISS to a 3% concentration.
4. Serum dilutions: dilute with buffered saline solution.

ONE-STAGE TEST

1. One drop of 3% red blood cell suspension.
2. One drop of serum or diluted serum.
3. Incubate the serum-cell mixture at 37 C for ten minutes.
4. Wash the red cells four times with normal saline solution.
5. Add two drops of antiglobulin serum to the tube-mix.
6. Centrifuge the tube for one minute at a low speed or for twenty-five seconds at 3,400 rpm.
7. Gently resuspend the red cell button and observe macroscopically for agglutination.
   Examine microscopically on a glass slide under low power.

TWO-STAGE TEST

1. One drop of 3% red cell suspension.
2. One drop of serum treated with 4 mg EDTA/ml.
3. Incubate serum-cell mixture at 37 C for five minutes.
4. Wash the cell four times with normal saline solution.
5. Add one volume of fresh normal AB or compatible serum to the bottom. Mix.
6. Incubate serum-cell mixture at 37 C for five minutes.
7. Centrifuge for twenty-four seconds at 3,400 rpm. Observe for hemolysis.
8. Wash the cells four times with normal saline solution.
9. Add two drops of anticomplement globulin serum.
10. Centrifuge for twenty-four seconds at 3,400 rpm.

11. Gently resuspend red cell button and observe macroscopically for agglutination. Examine microscopically on a slide under low power.

False positive reactions

Washing fresh or clotted red blood cells in LISS will cause the C4 and some C3 op-
ponents to attach to the red cells. An excess of the LISS may lower the ionic
strength below the optimal range of the serum and initiate the aggregation of serum
proteins, which in turn may cause the binding of C4 molecules to the red cells.
Bound complement components react with anti-C4 antibodies contained in a poly-
valent antihuman serum.

False negative reactions

Adding an excess of serum to the LISS suspended cells will raise the ionic strength
above the optimal range, and thus diminish the sensitivity of the procedure.

ABO BLOOD GROUPING

The ABO blood groups are determined by two separate procedures.

Direct Grouping

This consists of testing the unknown red cells against known anti-A, anti-B, and
anti-A, B (group O) antisera. This may be performed by the tube or the slide techniques. Freshly drawn anticoagulated or clotted blood specimens may be used, but
red cells properly preserved in ACD or Alsever's solution and stored at 4 C may be
tested for at least five days. The ABO blood groups are derived from an interpretation of the reactions observed as shown in Table 1.

Critique. Agglutination of the red cells will occur within seconds when potent antisera are used, except when some subgroups of A are encountered. The agglutination
of A_3, A_2B, and A_3B cells may occur more slowly with specific anti-A antisera used
in slide tests, but the routine use of anti-A, B (group O) antisera will detect the presence of these subgroups.

TABLE 1. INTERPRETATION FOR DIRECT GROUPING

Anti-A	Anti-B	Anti-A, B (group O)	Blood Group
+	−	+	A
−	+	+	B
+	+	+	AB
−	−	−	O

TABLE 2. INTERPRETATION FOR INDIRECT GROUPING

A₁ Cells	A₂ Cells	B Cells	O Cells	Blood Group
−	−	+	−	A
+	+	−	−	B
−	−	−	−	AB
+.	+	+	−	O

Indirect or Confirmatory Grouping

The serum of the individual who is being grouped for ABO is tested with known group A_1, B, and O red cells. When specific group A_1 cells are not available, a pool of three to five group A cells should be employed. The use of group A_2 cells is to be avoided since they can produce false negative results with weak anti-A antibodies. In addition, they will not detect anti-A_1 antibodies that may be present in the sera of some A_2 and A_2B individuals.

The results of this test are interpreted according to the scheme shown in Table 2. Before an ABO group can be assigned, the results of the direct and indirect groupings must show complete concordance.

This test is normally performed as a tube test, and occasionally hemolysis rather than agglutination will be observed. The presence of hemolysis is indicative of a positive reaction and is due to the complement in fresh serum. Hemolysis is not observed when plasma or serum that has been stored or inactivated is used for the confirmatory tests.

Testing for Subgroups of A

Characteristically, blood group A serum contains anti-B antibodies, and group AB serum is devoid of the primary blood group antibodies, but on occasion anti-A_1 antibodies are found in the serum of individuals of subgroups A_2, A_3, A_2B, and A_3B. Anti-A_1 antibodies are usually detected during confirmatory or indirect blood grouping. When they are found, it is important to identify the subgroup of A and AB, since in this situation specific group A_2 or A_2B blood must be used for transfusion.

The blood groups A and AB may be differentiated into subgroups A_1, A_2, A_3, A_1B, A_2B, or A_3B using slide or tube tests with either absorbed anti-A_1 serum or the anti-A_1 lectin (*Dolichos liflorus*). Supplementary tests may be performed with the anti-H lectin (*Ulex europeus*). Expected reactions in slide tests using anti-A_1 lectin are as follows:

1. Macroscopic agglutination of A_1 and A_1B red cells occurs within twenty to thirty seconds and is complete within one minute.
2. A_{int} red cells react more slowly, and moderate agglutination is noted at the end of one minute.
3. A_2 and A_2B red cells will not be agglutinated at the end of one minute. It is imperative that known A_1, A_2, and A_{int} red cell controls be incorporated

**TABLE 3. TUBE TEST REACTIONS OF A SUBGROUPS WITH ANTI-A₁
AND ANTI-H LECTINS**

	A_1	A_{int}	A_2	A_1B	A_2B	O	O_h (Bombay)
Anti-A₁ lectin	++++	+ to ++	−	++++	−	−	−
Anti-H lectin	−	++	++++	−	±	++++	−

For legend see Figure 1.

into the test system to check the validity of test results of the unknown red cells.

The expected results obtained in tube tests with anti-A₁ and anti-H lectins are given in Table 3.

Rh-Hr TYPING

The antigens of the Rh blood group system normally are detected using anti-Rh sera most reactive at 37 C that are designated for use either by the saline tube technique or by the slide/rapid tube method.

Slide/rapid tube reagents are used principally for Rh-Hr typing by the slide or "modified" test tube methods and for typing the D(Rh₀) variant, D^u.

Either clotted or anticoagulated red cells may be used to perform these determinations. The slide test requires a 40–50% concentration of red cells in plasma or serum. Blood specimens exhibiting low hematocrits are adjusted to the proper concentration by removing a portion of the serum or plasma. High concentrations of red cells in saline *cannot* be used for slide tests. If saline-suspended red cells are the only ones available, the cells must be centrifuged and the saline completely removed and replaced with normal human group AB serum.

The "modified" tube tests require a 2–4% suspension of red cells in the individual's own serum or in normal human group AB serum.

Autocontrols are necessary when one is performing both the slide and modified tube tests, since in vivo sensitized red cells from infants with hemolytic disease of the newborn and from patients with acquired hemolytic anemia or with red cells coated with abnormal macroglobulins may agglutinate spontaneously when exposed to the fortified Rh antisera.

Ideally, the autocontrols should be performed with the diluent the manufacturers used to prepare the antiserum. If this is not available, 22% bovine serum albumin can be used as a substitute. Red cells saturated with anti-Rh antibodies in vivo may fail to react with slide test Rh antisera, since the appropriate antigen sites on the red cells are blocked.

The general remarks pertaining to D(Rh₀) typing procedures apply to the detection of all the known Rh antigens (rh')C, (rh'')E, (Hr')c and (Hr'')e.

D(Rh$_o$) Slide Test

The slide test is the most popular procedure for rapid routine D(Rh$_o$) typing. It is performed as outlined in the general methods except that it is carried out on a viewing box prewarmed to 45–47 C by a light source and the test is observed for no more than two minutes. The temperature of the glass slide containing the serum-cell mixture reaches the ideal reaction temperature of 37–39 C when it is placed on the heated surface of the view box. It should be noted that it is not advisable to perform the Rh typings on the viewing box glass itself. Apart from this being poor laboratory technique, the elevated temperature will cause a rapid evaporation of the serum-red cell mixture, resulting in false positives, and the excessively high temperature can reduce or destroy the antibody activity of the antisera. Conversely, low temperatures increase the reaction time and false negatives will occur at the end of the two-minute test period.

Interpretation. The appearance of agglutination in the test system is indicative of the presence of the Rh antigen being tested for, provided that agglutination is absent in the autocontrols. Agglutination in the autocontrol invalidates the test and it must be repeated with the use of saline reactive reagents.

Sources of error. False positives may occur for a number of reasons, including:

1. Evaporation due to high temperature or prolonged incubation time (slide test).
2. Bacterial contamination of the red cells.
3. Heavy rouleaux formation (slide test).
4. Presence of autoagglutinins or in vivo sensitized red cells.

False negatives may occur as the result of:

1. Weak red cell suspensions (less than a 40% concentration in slide tests).
2. Improper mixture of the antiserum with the cells (slide test).
3. Hemolyzed red cells—old or bacterially contaminated cells.
4. Failure to maintain the viewing box at the 45–47 C temperatures (slide tests).
5. Use of antisera that have lost their reactivity because of outdating, bacterial contamination, or inadvertant dilution with human serum, saline, or bovine albumin.
6. Red cells of infants with hemolytic disease of the newborn due to saturation of the cells with anti-D antibody in vivo.
7. Failure to add the antiserum or the inadvertant addition of albumin to the drop of blood in place of the antiserum.

Modified Tube Test

The procedure is carried out as outlined in the general directions for tube tests with the exception that a 2–4% suspension of freshly prepared red cells in the patient's own serum, normal human group AB serum, or 20% bovine serum albumin is used and the test is incubated at 37 C.

Interpretation. As in the slide test, presence of agglutination in the antiserum tubes and absence in the autocontrol tubes indicate the presence of $D(Rh_o)$ antigen. Agglutination of the autocontrol invalidates the result and the tests must be repeated using saline active anti-$D(Rh_o)$ antisera. This is performed exactly as outlined in the general directions with the exception that the red cells must be washed and suspended in saline at a concentration of 2–4%.

Sources of error. False positive or negative reactions in tube tests may be encountered for the same reasons as for the slide tests.

Testing for Rh_o Variant (D^u)

Many anti-D antisera are capable of detecting the Rh_o variant (D^u) directly, although standard tests cannot be relied on exclusively for this purpose. Normally, the indirect antiglobulin test, a more sensitive method, is used to type this antigen. The test is carried out as outlined in the general directions for the indirect antiglobulin procedure and a potent incomplete anti-D antisera is used to sensitize the red cells. An autocontrol should be tested in parallel.

Interpretation. Agglutination of the red cells by the antiserum with a negative autocontrol variant indicates that D^u is present. Absence of agglutination indicates that D^u is absent.

ANTIBODY SCREENING AND IDENTIFICATION

1. Prepare and number four rows of 10×75 mm test tubes. The number of tubes required for each row is determined by the number of cells contained in the reagent red cell panel, the autocontrol. The number of rows may be increased if enzyme procedures are indicated or decreased if the available volume of serum is insufficient.
2. Prepare suspensions of washed reagent red cells as follows:
   For Row 1—Saline 22–25 C (room temperature).
   For Row 2—Saline 16 C.
   For Row 3—Saline 37 C.
   For Row 4—Bovine serum albumin 30–22%. When using 22% albumin, resuspend the red cells in normal human group AB serum.
3. Place two drops of the serum to be tested into each of the test tubes of each row.

4. Add one drop of the appropriate cell suspensions to the properly numbered tube of serum in each row or one drop of a 2–4% serum suspension of red cells to the fourth row when 22% albumin is used.
5. Add either three drops of 30% albumin or two drops of 22% albumin to each tube in row four. Mix the contents thoroughly.
6. Centrifuge rows three and four separately. The saline row (three) will normally require half as much centrifugation as the albumin row (four).
7. Observe both rows for hemolysis. Then gently resuspend the cell buttons and observe for macroscopic agglutination. Caution must be exercised in observing for hemolysis of the test cells, since hemolysis is not encountered with the regularity of agglutination.
8. Record the degree of hemolysis and/or agglutination.
9. Incubate rows one, two, three, and four at their respective temperatures for one hour.
10. Centrifuge each row separately and record the results.
11. Perform an indirect antiglobulin test on each of the tubes in rows three and four according to the method previously described, beginning at the wash step.
12. Centrifuge rows one and two to produce clearly defined red cell buttons and return the test tubes to their respective temperatures for five to ten minutes.
13. Gently resuspend the cell buttons and record the degree of hemolysis and/or agglutination of each tube.
    (Note: Fresh active serum should be used in this test. If the serum is old or has been contaminated with bacteria, an additional tube for each cell must be used. This should contain one drop of 3% cells in fresh normal AB serum as a source of complement, and two drops of serum to be tested. These tubes are incubated at 37 C for thirty minutes and the antiglobulin test is then performed.)
14. The reactions of the unknown serum are then compared with the alloantigenic mosaic of the cells in the panel. The positive and negative reactions should make it possible to identify the unknown antibody.

    If no known specificity corresponds to that of the unknown, four things must be considered: a. The unknown serum contains a mixture of antibodies; b. the antibody involved is detecting an antigen for which the panel has not been tested; c. the cells in the panel are exhibiting dosage effects; and d. the antibody is detecting a completely new antigenic determinant. Further studies, including absorption and elution procedures, must be considered.

COMPATIBILITY TESTING

The compatibility test, or direct cross-match, normally consists of three phases performed simultaneously: a saline test, a high protein test, and an indirect antiglobulin test.

Saline Cross-Match

1. Place two drops of the recipient's serum into an appropriately labeled 10 × 75 mm test tube.
2. Add one drop of 2–4% saline suspension of the donor's red cells.
3. Incubate the tubes at room temperature for thirty minutes.
4. Centrifuge.
5. Gently resuspend the cell buttons and observe macroscopically for agglutination.

High Protein Cross-Match (30% Bovine Serum Albumin)

1. Prepare a 2–4% suspension of the donor's red cells in saline.
2. Place two drops of the recipient's serum into appropriately marked tubes.
3. Add one drop of a 2–4% saline suspension of the donor's red cells.
4. Add three drops of 30% bovine serum albumin.
5. Mix well and centrifuge immediately at the rate of speed previously determined for a variable or a fixed-speed centrifuge. Immediate centrifugation will prevent a prozone effect when a serum contains a high titer of antibodies.
6. Resuspend the red cell button gently and observe for macroscopic agglutination.
7. If agglutination is absent, incubate at 37 C for thirty minutes.
8. Centrifuge and examine red cell buttons for agglutination.

INDIRECT ANTIGLOBULIN CROSS-MATCH

1. Place two drops of the recipient's serum or plasma in an appropriately labeled 10 × 75 mm test tube.
2. Add one drop of a 2–4% saline suspension of the donor's red cells. Mix both tubes thoroughly.
3. Incubate at 37 C for thirty minutes.
4. Wash the incubated red cell serum mixture three times with saline.
5. Decant the saline completely after the last washing to secure "dry buttons."
6. Resuspend the cell button with the saline that remains on the interfaces of the test tubes.
7. Add two drops of antiglobulin serum to each test tube. Mix thoroughly.
8. Centrifuge.
9. Gently resuspend the cell buttons and observe macroscopically for agglutination. A hand lens or a magnifying reading mirror may be used to read the weaker reactions.

Interpretation. A smooth suspension of red cells in all cross-match phases indicates that the donor's blood is compatible for infusing the recipient. Agglutination in any phase is indicative of an incompatible direct matching procedure.

Specialized Procedures

ENZYME TREATMENT OF RED CELLS

Trypsin[3]

1. Stock solution: 1 gm trypsin powder 1:250.
   100 ml phosphate buffer pH 7.3 [76.8 ml $Na_2HPO_42H_2O$ (0.1188% in H_2O) + 23.2 ml Kh_2PO_4 (0.0908% in H_2O)].
2. Wash red cells three times and prepare a 2% saline suspension.
3. Add one part of stock trypsin solution to nine parts of the cell suspension.
4. Incubate for ten minutes in a 37C water bath.
5. Wash three times with ice cold saline and reconstitute to the original volume with saline. The cell suspension is now ready for use.

Ficin[4]

1. Stock solution: 1 gm ficin (use extreme caution when handling this material).
   100 ml physiologic saline.
   Working solution: One part of stock solution plus nine parts of Hendry's buffer. [1 part NaH_2PO_4 (0.514% in H_2O) + 4 parts Na_2HPO_4 (0.445% in H_2O)].
2. Wash red cells three times and prepare a 50% suspension in saline.
3. Mix equal volumes of cell suspension and the working solution of ficin.
4. Incubate for fifteen minutes in a 37C water bath.

5. Wash twice with physiologic saline and adjust the cell concentration to 2% in saline. The cells are now ready for use.

Papain[5]

1. Papain solution:
   a. 2 gm papain 1:350.
      100 ml M/15 phosphate buffer pH 5.4 [964 ml KH_2PO_4 (0.0908% in H_2O) + 36 ml $Na_2HPO_42H_2O$ (0.1188% in H_2O)].
   b. Filter stock solution and add 10 ml M/2 cysteine (7.9% L-cysteine HCl in H_2O).
   c. Dilute to 200 ml with buffer.
   d. Incubate sixty minutes in a 37C water bath.
   e. Dispense in small tubes and freeze at −20C. The solution is stable for about four months.
2. Mix three volumes of enzyme solution with one volume of antiserum or, if the antiserum is weak, use equal volumes.
3. Place 0.1 ml of enzyme-antiserum mixture into a 10 × 75 mm test tube.
4. Add 0.1 ml of a 3% suspension of red cells in saline.
5. Mix and incubate for two hours in a 37C water bath.
6. Observe macroscopically without centrifugation.

Bromelin[6]

1. Stock solution: 0.5% bromelin in nine parts saline and one part phosphate buffer, pH 5.5 [0.35 volumes of M/15 Na_2HPO_4 (9.46 gm per liter) to 9.65 volumes of M/15 KH_2PO_4 (9.07 gm per liter)].
2. Add one drop of stock bromelin solution to 0.1 ml of serum and one drop of a 4% suspension of red cells.
3. Incubate at 37C for fifteen minutes.
4. Centrifuge at 1,000 rpm for one minute.
5. Observe macroscopically for agglutination (Fig. 1).

ANTIBODY TITRATION

The titer, or relative amount of antibodies is determined by testing serial dilutions of the serum.

1. Wash a quantity of group O test red cells bearing the appropriate antigen three times to remove all traces of plasma and free hemoglobin. Red cells requiring more than three washings to eliminate the evidence of hemolysis are unfit for use, and new samples of test cells should be obtained.

2. Prepare an exact 2% suspension of cells in saline and 20 or 22% albumin diluents by adding 0.2 ml of washed, packed, tested cells to 9.8 ml of the suspending medium—saline or albumin.

Saline-Antiglobulin Titration

Use a clean 0.2 ml pipette for each transfer to avoid serum "carry-over" from previous tube.

1. Label twelve test tubes (10 × 75 mm) with the dilution of the serum each tube will contain: 1, 2, 4, 8, 16, 32, 64, 128, 256, 512, 1024, and C.
2. Add 0.1 ml of saline to tubes two through C.
3. Add 0.1 ml of the serum to be titrated to tubes 1 and 2.
4. Beginning with tube two, mix well, and transfer 0.1 ml of the diluted serum to tube four.
5. Continue the transfers until a dilution of 1:1024 is reached. The C tube is a diluent control and receives no antibody. Do not discard the extra 0.1 ml in the tube, since it may be useful if higher dilutions of the serum are needed to complete the titration procedure.
6. Add 0.1 ml of the exact 2% saline suspension of red cells to each tube, one through C.
7. Shake the serum mixture well.
8. Incubate at 37C for sixty minutes.
9. Centrifuge the tubes.
10. Observe for hemolysis and/or agglutination.
11. Wash all tubes three times with saline.
12. Add two drops of antiglobulin antiserum to each washed tube.
13. Centrifuge the washed tubes.
14. Observe for agglutination. Score the agglutination reactions. The titer of an antibody is the reciprocal of the highest dilution in which a full 1+ agglutination reaction is recorded.

Albumin-Antiglobulin Titration

1. Wash the test cells three times with normal saline solution or spin down the 2% saline suspension of red cells.
2. Resuspend the packed red cells in 20 or 22% albumin to a 2% suspension.
3. Dilute the serum by substituting either 20 or 22% albumin, or neutral AB serum for the saline diluent.
4. Incubate at 37C for one hour.
5. Centrifuge.
6. Gently resuspend the cell buttons. Score the agglutination reactions the same as for the saline-antiglobulin methods.

Pitfalls in Titration Procedures

1. The red cell suspensions should be prepared and used immediately, since cells suspended in saline and albumin for an indefinite period of time will hemolyze. Titrations with hemolyzed suspensions of red cells will be worthless.
2. Each tube in the dilution series must be examined before a serum is considered to be negative, since the first several tubes may be negative because of the prozone phenomenon.

ABSORPTION OF ANTISERUM

1. Inactivate the serum in a 56C water bath for thirty minutes.
2. Add an equal volume of heat-inactivated serum to washed packed cells from which the supernatant has been removed as completely as possible.
3. Incubate for fifteen minutes with continuous agitation. The incubation temperature depends on the type of antibodies being absorbed, i.e., incomplete antibodies would be absorbed at 37C, complete antibodies at room temperature, and cold agglutinins at 4C.
4. Centrifuge for ten minutes at 3,000 rpm.
5. Remove the supernatant for testing.
6. Repeat the absorption with fresh aliquots of cells until a fresh suspension of the cells being used for absorption is no longer agglutinated by the serum under the conditions used in the test.

ELUTION OF ANTIBODIES FROM RED CELLS—CLASSICAL METHOD[7]

1. Wash the sensitized cells four times with saline at 4C.
2. Pack the cells by centrifugation for ten minutes at 3,000 rpm.
3. Resuspend the cells in one-third their volume of either saline or 6% bovine albumin: 6% bovine albumin is better for red cell testing; saline is better for immunoglobulin analysis.
4. Place in a 56 C water bath for ten minutes with constant agitation.
5. Rapidly centrifuge in preheated centrifuge cups at 3,000 rpm for one minute.
6. Draw off the supernatant fluid containing the eluate immediately. (Note: Eluates should always be tested on the day of their preparation.)

RAPID ACID-STROMAL ELUTION METHOD
(Adapted from Jenkins and Moore[8])

Reagents:

1. Physiologic saline solution 0.145 M. (8.5 gm NaCl in 1,000 ml H_2O).
2. Digitonin suspension 5 mgm/ml (2.5 gm digitonin in 500 ml physiologic saline. Shake thoroughly before using to insure a uniform suspension.)
3. 0.1 M glycine-HCl buffer pH 3.0 (7.5 gm glycine in 800 ml H_2O. Adjust to pH 3.0 by adding 1.0 N HCl gradually. q.s. to 1,000 ml with distilled water. Store at 4 C to insure stability).
4. 0.8M K_2NaPO_4 buffer pH 8.2 (0.8 M K_2HPO_4 − 95 volumes + 0.8 M NaH_2PO_4 − 5 volumes)

1. Wash the antibody-coated red blood cells three times with saline.
2. To 1.0 ml of the washed packed cells add 9.0 ml of saline. Resuspend the red cells (10% red cell suspension).
3. Add 0.5 ml of the digitonin solution.
4. Allow the red cells to completely hemolyze, which usually takes two to three minutes for complete hemolysis.
5. Centrifuge at 3,400 rpm for five minutes.
6. Discard the supernatant solution.
7. Wash the red cell stroma with saline until the supernatant is clear, usually at least three times.
8. Add 2.0 ml glycine HCl to the packed stroma. Mix well.
9. Allow to stand for one minute at room temperature.
10. Centrifuge at 3,400 rpm for five minutes.
11. Remove the supernatant solution to a clean test tube.
12. Add 0.2 ml of the K_2NaPO_4 buffer to the supernatant solution immediately to prevent denaturation of the antibodies at pH 3.0.
13. Centrifuge at 3,400 rpm for five minutes to clear any precipitate that may form.
14. Remove the supernatant solution, which is the eluate. The final pH of the supernatant is 7.0–7.2.
15. Test the eluate for antibody activity.

LYMPHOCYTE
MICROCYTOTOXICITY—TWO-STAGE METHOD
(Adapted from Mittal et al.[9])

Lymphocyte Suspension—Ficoll method adapted from Terasaki[10]

1. Collect 10 ml of blood and mix with 0.1 of heparin (5,000 units per ml USP; *phenol free*).

2. Centrifuge the whole blood for five minutes at 3,000 rpm in a swinging bucket rotor.
3. Remove 2 ml of buffy coat and divide between two Fisher tubes. Centrifuge for two minutes in the Model 59 Fisher centrifuge at 2,000 g.
4. Remove the buffy coat, avoiding as many red cells as possible, and place into a 16 × 100 mm test tube containing five drops of anti-A, B, or anti-H and three drops of adenosine diphosphate (ADP: 1 mg/ml).
5. Gently rotate the tube for two to five minutes to agglutinate the red cells and platelets.
6. Transfer the mixture to a Fisher tube and centrifuge for three seconds at 1,000 g.
7. Remove the supernatant and layer over 0.4 ml of Ficoll-Hypaque (R.I. 1.3530) contained in each of two Fisher tubes and centrifuge for two minutes at 1,000 g.
8. Transfer the white interface containing the lymphocytes into a clear Fisher tube and wash twice with IX Hanks solution.
9. Resuspend the cells in the desired media and adjust the concentration.

Test procedure

1. The test is carried out in Falcon plastic microtissue culture trays (Falcon Plastics, Los Angeles, California).
2. Fill the wells in the tray with extra heavy mineral oil.
3. Dispense 1 μl of antiserum into each well.
4. Add 1 μl of lymphocyte suspension to each well. Care must be taken to ensure that the suspension is added directly into the antiserum.
5. Incubate for thirty minutes at room temperature.
6. Add 5 μl of rabbit complement to each test and incubate for one hour at room temperature.
7. Add 2 μl of rabbit complement to each test and incubate for one hour at room temperature.
8. Add 2 μl of 40% neutralized formalin (pH 7.0). Neutralized formalin: 500 ml formaldehyde; 0.5 gm of $NaH_2PO_4H_2O$; 1.5 gm Na_2HPO_4.
9. Read the tests on an inverted microscope under phase contrast illumination at a magnification of 150X. Reading is simplified if a 3″ × 4″ glass cover slide is placed over the wells just prior to reading. Under these conditions living lymphocytes exhibit a glowing appearance, with little or no nuclear detail. Dead cells appear swollen, with dark prominent nuclei.
10. The test is graded as follows:

% OF CELL DEATH	GRADE	INTERPRETATION
0 to 10	1	Negative
10 to 25	2	Questionable
25 to 50	4	Weak positive
50 to 80	6	Positive
80 to 100	8	Strong positive

REFERENCES

1. Renton PH and Hancock JA: Anti-body-like effects of colloidal silica. Vox Sang 2:117, 1957.
2. Moore HC and Mollison PL: Use of low-ionic strength medium in manual tests for antibody detection. Transfusion 16:291, 1976.
3. Morton JA and Pickles MM: Use of trypsin in the detection of incomplete anti-Rh antibodies. Nature 159:779, 1947.
4. Haber G and Rosenfield RE: Ficin treated red cells for hemagglutination studies. P. H. Andresen Festkrift. Copenhagen, Munksgaard, 1957.
5. Low B: A practical method using papain and incomplete Rh-antibodies in routine Rh blood grouping. Vox Sang 5:94, 1955.
6. Mollison PL: Blood Transfusion in Clinical Medicine. 4th ed. Philadelphia, F. A. Davis, 1967.
7. Landsteiner K and Miller CP Jr: Serological studies on the blood of primates. II. The blood groups in anthropoid apes. J Exp Med 42:853, 1925.
8. Jenkins DE Jr and Moore WH: A rapid method for the preparation of high potency auto- and alloantibodies. Transfusion 17:110, 1977.
9. Mittal KK, Mickey MR, Singal DP, and Terasaki PI: Serotyping for homotransplantation. XVIII. Refinement of microdroplet lymphocyte cytotoxicity test. Transplantation 6:913, 1968.
10. Terasaki PI and Park MS: Microdroplet lymphocytotoxicity test. NIAID Manual of Tissue Typing Techniques, DHEW Publication No. 80-545 (NIH). Washington, DC, 1979, pp 92–103.

Papers of Historical Significance
On Agglutination of Normal Human Blood*

Karl Landsteiner
Assistant at the Pathological-Anatomical Institute, Vienna

The following contains a collection of historically significant classical papers documenting the original description of the ABO, MN, and Rh blood groups. They have been reprinted with the kind permission of the original publishers and are included not only as a source of information but, more importantly, for the sake of enjoyment. It is truly refreshing to experience the beautiful simplicity with which the keen observations of prepared and unclouded minds led to the fundamental knowledge that forms the basis of contemporary blood-grouping science.

Some time ago I observed and reported that serum of normal humans frequently agglutinates red blood cells of other healthy individuals.[1] At that time I was under the impression that this ability of the serum to agglutinate foreign red cells was especially pronounced in some diseases and I believed that this agglutinating ability was related to the strong lytic ability of pathologic sera on normal red cells which was observed by Maragliano[2] many years ago. This concept seemed to be supported by the fact that agglutinating and lytic abilities frequently, although not always, changed in a parallel fashion. However, the fact that the addition of sodium chloride up to normal concentrations will (although heating will not) destroy this lytic ability of the sera indicates the reactions of Maragliano are not identical to the hemolytic reactions of the blood sera which are being investigated so intensively. Maragliano himself differentiates his observations from the phenomenon of Landois-hemolysis caused by foreign serum, since in Maragliano's case hemoglobin is not only dissolved but also destroyed. A fundamental difference between my ob-

* Translated from the original German, which appeared in Wiener Klinische Wochenschrift 14:1132 (1901), by Professor A. L. Kappus, Chairman of the Department of Microbiology at the Marquette University School of Medicine, and reprinted from Transfusion 1:5 (1961) with permission of J. B. Lippincott Co., Philadelphia, PA.

servations and those of Maragliano is that in his case the serum acts also upon the red blood cells of the same individual and that his reaction occurs with pathologic blood only. My observations, however, reveal characteristic differences between blood serum and red blood cells of various apparently healthy persons.

The report and pictures presented by Shattock[3] describe a related phenomenon, although he found the reaction only in febrile diseases and failed to see it with normal blood. Shattock thinks that the reaction is connected with the increased coagulability and rouleaux formation of the febrile blood.

The agglutination of human blood by human serum ought to be called isoagglutination according to the nomenclature of Ehrlich and Morgenroth. Shortly after my publication these two investigators reported experiments in which they injected blood of the same species and thereby succeeded in preparing isoagglutinins and isolysins, that is, sera which act upon the red blood cells of the same species. These very comprehensive experiments confirm the unexpected existence of clearly demonstrable differences between the bloods within one animal species.

In the paper of Ehrlich and Morgenroth[4] the phenomena of isolysis are discussed in regard to the theoretical concepts presented by Ehrlich.

Since the publication of the reports of Shattock and myself a number of investigators studied isoagglutination in man. The fact that the reaction occurs in the blood of healthy individuals renders those papers valueless which consider the reaction specific for certain diseases.[5] Other papers even report observations concerning the intensity and frequency of the reaction in diseases.

Donath[6] found the reaction more frequently in patients with different forms of anemia than in healthy people, though this was not always the case. Ascoli[7] observed the reaction in healthy individuals but noted greater intensity in diseased ones. Eisenberg investigated healthy and diseased persons. He, like others, came to the conclusion that the reaction occurs frequently in diseased but only exceptionally in healthy persons. This, however, contradicts my statements.[8]

As I have given only a very brief report in my paper mentioned above I would like to present the results of some recent experiments. The tables need no interpretation. Equal amounts of serum and of 5 per cent red blood cell suspension in 0.6 percent sodium chloride were mixed and observed in a hanging drop preparation or in the test tube. (The + sign signifies agglutination.)

A fourth similar table concerning the sera of Table 2 mixed with the red blood cells of Table 1 and some other tested sera, for instance those of one case of hemo-

TABLE 1. CONCERNING THE BLOOD OF SIX APPARENTLY HEALTHY MEN

Sera						
Dr. St.	−	+	+	+	−	
Dr. Plecn.	−	−	+	+	−	−
Dr. Sturl.	−	+	−	−	+	−
Dr. Erdh.	−	+	−	−	+	−
Zar.	−	−	+	+	−	−
Landst.	−	+	+	+	+	−
Rbc's of:	Dr. St.	Dr. Plecn.	Dr. Sturl.	Dr. Erdh.	Zar.	Landst.

TABLE 2. CONCERNING THE BLOOD OF SIX APPARENTLY HEALTHY PUERPERAL WOMEN

Sera						
Scil.	−	−	+	−	−	+
Linsm.	+	−	+	+	+	+
Lust.	+	−	−	+	+	−
Mittlelb.	−	−	+	−	−	+
Tomsch.	−	−	+	−	−	+
Graupn.	+	−	−	+	+	−
Rbc's of:	Scil.	Linsm.	Lust.	Mettelb.	Tomsch.	Graupn.

TABLE 3. CONCERNING THE BLOOD OF FIVE PUERPERAL AND SIX PLACENTAE (CORD BLOOD)

Sera						
Lust.	+	+	−	−	−	+
Tomsch.	−	−	+	−	−	−
Mittelb.	−	−	+	−	−	−
Seil.	−	−	+	−	−	−
Linsm.	+	+	+	−	−	+
Rbc's of:	Trautm.	Linsm.	Seil.	Freib.	Graupn.	Mittelb.

philia and one case of purpura, presents entirely identical regularities and is therefore omitted. The investigation of another ten normal persons (in 42 combinations) gave similar results.

These experiments prove that I do not have to correct my statement. The reaction was given by all of the 22 tested sera from healthy adults. Obviously, this result would not have been obtained if I had not used a number of different red blood cells for the test.

Halban,[9] Ascoli, and finally Eisenberg have already reported on the variable resistance of red blood cells towards the reaction. This is also shown in the above tables. Moreover, there was a peculiar regularity in the reaction of the 22 tested blood specimens. If one disregards some tests with sera from fetal placental blood which do not cause agglutination—Halban also found fetal blood serum rarely agglutinates—the sera may, in most cases, be grouped in three groups.

In a number of cases (Group A) the serum reacts with the red blood cells of another group (B) but not with the red blood cells of Group A; these react with the serum B in an identical way. In the third group C the serum agglutinates the red blood cells of Group A and B but the red blood cells of C are not influenced by the sera of A and B.

Applying the commonly used technical terms it may be said that there exist at least two different types of agglutinins, one in A, another one in B, and both together in C. The red blood cells are inert to the agglutinins which are present in the same serum.

No doubt a report concerning the presence of a few different agglutinins in the cases tested sounds peculiar, although the experiments of Ehrlich and Morgenroth with isolysins showed quite similar conditions; it might be more satisfactory to find another interpretation by further observation.

It is suggested that attention be paid to these regularities in pathological cases.

Eisenberg thinks that the production of agglutinins is due to the resorption of components of red blood cells. This idea is not new; Halban and Ascoli have already presented it as a possible explanation. I did not formerly refer to it because I did not succeed in producing autoagglutination by injecting animals with their own lysed red blood cells.

I believe that Ehrlich does not report any positive results in that line either; Ascoli on the other hand obtained positive but not constant results. The difficulties of the given interpretation are mentioned by Halban. Perhaps the origin of naturally occurring hemagglutinins and normal agglutinins reacting with bacteria require different explanations.

Furthermore, my experiments show that various sera do not act identically as far as agglutination is concerned. Thus, if one believes that their agglutinating ability is developed in response to some autoimmunization due to resorption of cell components one has also to assume individual differences in order to interpret different sera. Actually, there are differences in different red blood cells and even already in fetal blood. Even if one acknowledges the differences of the sera or the red blood cells, the agglutination within species is just as easy or as difficult to understand as the agglutination by a serum from another species.

Nonetheless the presented interpretation cannot be disregarded; it is even the most adequate one if the untested experiments of Ascoli are correct. Then the physiological disintegration of the cells of body tissues might well be responsible for the formation of active serum components.

The experiments with sera from infants and animals are well suited to exclude the influence of pathological processes which may have occurred in the past. Halban's experiments also provide evidence against such a relation.

The agglutination described can be performed with serum which is dried and promptly dissolved; I succeeded in obtaining it with blood dried on cotton cloth and dissolved after fourteen days. Provided rapid changes in the agglutinating ability do not occur the reaction may be suited to establish the identity, or more correctly the non-identity, of a blood specimen. In a second test, the six sera of Table 1 gave the same reaction as a fresh specimen obtained nine days previously.[10]

Finally, it might be mentioned that the reported observations may assist in the explanation of various consequences of therapeutical blood transfusions.

REFERENCES

1. Centralblatt für Bacteriologie XXVII. 8:361, v. 10. Februar 1900.
2. XI Congress für innere Medicin. Leipzig. 1892.
3. Journ. of Pathol. and Bacteriology. Februar 1900.
4. Berliner klinische Wochenschrift, 1900.
5. Literatur siehe bei Eisenberg, Wiener klinische Wochenschrift, 1901, Nr. 42.

6. Wiener klinische Wochenschrift, 1900, Nr. 22.
7. Münchener medicinische, 1901, S. 1229.
8. Although Eisenberg attacks my report in his paper, and at the same time confirms it in regard to the blood of patients, he mentions my paper in the bibliography but with no word in his text.
9. Wiener klinische Wochenschrift, 1900, Nr. 24.
10. Dr. Richter and I plan to investigate the reliability of this method.

A New Agglutinable Factor Differentiating Individual Human Bloods*

Karl Landsteiner and Philip Levine

From the Laboratories of the Rockefeller Institute for Medical Research

By absorbing a number of anti-human blood immune sera from rabbits with the blood corpuscles of certain individuals regardless of the group, fluids were obtained from a few sera which give a sharp differentiation of individual human bloods within the common blood groups.

Among 116 individuals selected from the four blood groups the distribution of the agglutinable factor (which may be designated as M) was as shown in Table II.

This reaction is distinguished by its intensity from some others known to show individual differences within the groups, such as the reactions with cold agglutinins.

This is a preliminary report.

* Reprinted from Proc Soc Exper Biol Med 24:600 (1927) with permission of The Society for Experimental Biology and Medicine, New York, NY

TABLE I.

Bloods	Serum No. 1020 diluted 1:20, absorbed with human blood, P.L. (Group II.)
J.K.	0
S.A.	++
D.F.	+++
L.S.	++
W.F.	++
W.D.	+++
P.L.	0
A.R.	++
E.J.	0
A.J.	+++
M.R.	++
S.M.	+
A.S.	++
H.S.	0
F.C.	++
H.G.	+++

Technic: 2 gtts. absorbed serum.
1 gtt. saline.
1 gtt. 2.5 per cent blood suspension.

TABLE II.

		White	Colored
Group I }	+	14	15
	0	2	5
Group II }	+	20	12
	0	3	5
Group III }	+	15	10
	0	4	4
Group IV }	+	4	1
	0	2	0
Total number		64	
Total positive		53	
Total negative		11	

Further Observations on Individual Differences of Human Blood*

Karl Landsteiner and Philip Levine

From the Laboratories of the Rockefeller Institute for Medical Research

In a previous communication[1] we described an agglutinable factor (M), independent of the blood groups and present in many but not in all human bloods. A somewhat higher incidence of M among colored than white individuals, as indicated by our first results, was confirmed by examination on a larger scale; among 902 white individuals 165 (18.3 per cent), and among 338 colored 95 (28.1 per cent) whose blood reacted negatively. A differentiation of bloods (in the same group) lacking or possessing the factor M, was possible also with dried specimens.

The heredity of the property M was studied in more than 100 families. The results are in keeping with the assumption that M is inherited as a mendelian dominant. In the following table the families are arranged in 3 classes according to the presence or absence of the factor M in the parents, and its incidence among the offspring is given.

It may be mentioned incidentally that the character[2] A^1 present in most bloods of group A, seems to be an inheritable quality. For, in our tests, if the property was not or slightly developed in the blood of both parents, this, as a rule, was also the case for the children.

With a method similar to that employed for the detection of M, namely, suitable adsorption of certain rabbit immune sera for human blood, two other agglutinable qualities were found which may be denoted as N and P. These reactions, further distinguishing individual human bloods, vary in intensity from very strong to weak or negative.

The reactions for N seem to be strong in most cases where M is absent. The

---

* Reprinted from Proc Soc Exper Biol Med 24:941–942 (1927)
[1] Landsteiner, K., and Levine, P., Proc. Soc. Exp. Biol. and Med., 1927, xxiv, 600.
[2] For the terminology see Landsteiner, K., and Witt, D.H., J. of Immunol., 1926, xi, 221.

property M could be demonstrated also in the blood of eight chimpanzees examined, but was not found in the blood of five gibbons.

Strong reactions for P were considerably more frequent with the blood of colored than white individuals; similar results were also obtained with suitably absorbed normal rabbit and horse sera.

TABLE 1

Number of families	65		39		3	
Parents	+	+	+	−	−	−
Number of children	252+	25−	114+	52−	0+	11−

An Unusual Case of Intra-Group Agglutination*

Philip Levine and Rufus E. Stetson

From the Department of Laboratories, Newark Beth Israel
Hospital, Newark, NJ and The Blood Transfusion
Betterment Association of New York City

This report deals with a rare property in the blood of a patient whose serum showed an iso-agglutinin of moderate activity, which agglutinated about 80 per cent of the bloods of her own group. In view of the fact that this agglutinin tended to disappear after an interval of several months and the fact that this agglutinin gave an equally strong reaction at 37 and 20 C., it would seem to resemble agglutinins resulting from iso-immunization following repeated transfusions. This phenomenon is readily reproduced in some species (cattle, chickens, rabbits), by several repeated transfusions, but in the case of man only two clear-cut instances of such iso-immunization to cellular elements are described in the literature.[1] The case to be described differs from these in that the immune iso-agglutinin must have been stimulated by a factor other than repeated transfusion. The nature of this factor becomes evident from a summary of the case history.

REPORT OF CASE

M. S., a woman aged 25, a secundipara, was registered in the antepartum clinic of Bellevue Hospital July 12, 1937, at which time she showed some pretibal edema and a blood pressure of 130 systolic, 90 diastolic. (The expected date of delivery was in the last week of October.) Two weeks later the blood pressure was 154 systolic, 106 diastolic, and there was a faint trace of albumin in the urine. Hospitalization and rest in bed resulted in subsidence of all symptoms. The fetal heart sounds were not heard, but there were no x-ray signs of fetal death.

Labor pains and vaginal bleeding started on September 8 (the thirty-third

* Reprinted from JAMA 113:126 (1939) with permission of the publishers and the authors.

week of the gestation), and at midnight September 9 the patient was admitted to the hospital, at which time labor pains lasting one minute occurred every five minutes. There was considerable bleeding before the membranes were ruptured, and a macerated stillborn fetus weighing only 1 pound 5 ounces (595 Gm.) was delivered. After the placenta was expelled, bleeding was finally controlled and the patient (group O) was given her first transfusion of 500 cc. of whole blood from her husband (group O). Ten minutes after she received the blood a chill developed and she complained of pains in her legs and head. About twelve hours later a piece of membrane was passed and this was followed by more bleeding. At 4 p. m. a second transfusion of 750 cc. of whole blood was given, apparently without any reactions. In view of the renewed bleeding, hysterectomy was performed, followed by a third transfusion of 800 cc. of whole blood with no reaction.

Nineteen hours after the first transfusion and eight hours after the hysterectomy the patient voided 8 ounces (240 cc.) of bloody and dusky urine. At this time tests done with a more delicate technic revealed that, although the patient and her husband—the first donor whose blood caused a reaction—were in group O, the patient's serum nevertheless agglutinated distinctly her husband's cells and, indeed, the cells of most group O donors. Subsequently the patient received six more uneventful transfusions from compatible professional donors very carefully selected by the Blood Transfusion Betterment Association.

Subsequent intensive treatment—diathermy over the kidneys, forced fluids by vein, rectum and mouth, the repeated transfusions mentioned and high hot colonic irrigations—resulted in gradual recovery of kidney function.

COMMENT

The blood was referred to us during the patient's convalescence, October 9, a month after the hysterectomy. Tests previously performed at the Donor Bureau of the Blood Transfusion Betterment Association showed that only eight of fifty group O donors did not react with the patient's serum and hence were compatible. In our series of fifty-four bloods of group O, thirteen failed to react with the patient's serum. Thus, of a total of 104 group O bloods twenty-one were compatible.

It could be readily shown that these reactions differ from those due to so-called atypical agglutinins occasionally found in the serums of normal persons. The former reactions were just as active at 37 as at 20 C., while reactions of the latter variety as a rule do not occur at 37 C. or else are considerably diminished. In other words, identical results were obtained when tests with serums of the patient were kept either at 20 or at 37 C. or were read after centrifuging and resuspending the sedimented cells.

The reactions were found to be independent of the M, N or P blood factors. Owing to the lack of suitable quantities of the blood, it was not possible to perform absorption experiments in order to supply data on the incidence of the reactions in bloods of groups A, B and AB.

Another specimen drawn two months later, December 3, still exhibited the agglutinin, which however gave far weaker reactions. Here again the reactions at 37 C. were just as intense as those at room temperature or lower. It was not possible to examine the serum of this patient until a year later, when all traces of reactions had disappeared.

In several respects this iso-agglutinin, as already mentioned, resembles the iso-agglutinins described by Landsteiner, Levine and Janes and that of Neter, namely (1) reactions within the same group equally active at room temperature and at 37C. and (2) the temporary character of the agglutinin. In both of these cases the agglutinin was not demonstrable until an interval of several weeks had elapsed following repeated transfusions. In the present case, however, it is evident that the unusual iso-agglutinin must have been present at the time the patient was given her first transfusion with the blood of her husband, which subsequently was shown to be sensitive. Furthermore, this first transfusion was not uneventful in view of the resulting chills, pains in the legs and intense headache.

It is well established that in instances of iso-immunization in animals the iso-agglutinin serves as a reagent to detect dominant hereditary blood factors in the red blood cells and presumably also in the tissue cells. In view of the fact that this patient harbored a dead fetus for a period of several months, one may assume that the products of the disintegrating fetus were responsible not only for the toxic symptoms of the patient but also for the iso-immunization. Presumably the immunizing property in the blood and/or tissues of the fetus must have been inherited from the father. Since this dominant property was not present in the mother, specific immunization conceivably could occur.

No data are available as to the relationship to one another of the immune iso-agglutinin in the two previously reported cases and in the present case. Judging from the frequency of positive and negative reactions, it is evident that the iso-agglutinin in this case is distinct from the other two; i.e., 20 per cent nonreacting bloods in contrast with 75 per cent in the case of Neter and 60 per cent in that of Landsteiner, Levine and Janes.

Agglutinins of this sort can rarely be investigated thoroughly because of their tendency to diminish in activity and eventually to disappear. Consequently, attempts were made to produce a hetero-immune agglutinin of identical or similar specificity by repeated injections of sensitive blood into a series of rabbits. These experiments met with failure, since suitable absorption tests with such serums failed to reveal the presence of the desired agglutinin.

REFERENCE

1. Landsteiner, Karl, Levine, Philip, and Janes, M.L.: Proc. Soc. Exper. Biol. & Med. 25:672 (May) 1928. Neter, Erwin: J. Immunol. 30:255 (March) 1936.

An Agglutinable Factor in Human Blood Recognized by Immune Sera for Rhesus Blood*

Karl Landsteiner and Alexander S. Wiener

From the Rockefeller Institute for Medical Research and the Office of the Chief Medical Examiner of New York City

The capacity possessed by some rabbit immune sera produced with blood of Rhesus monkeys, of reacting with human bloods that contain the agglutinogen M has been reported previously.[1,2] Subsequently it has been found that another individual property of human blood (which may be designated as Rh) can be detected by certain of these sera.

Upon exhaustion of such a serum with selected bloods, for instance OM, the absorbed serum still agglutinated the majority (39 out of 45) of other human bloods, independently of the group or the M, N type; moreover, reactions took place with bloods lacking the property P. An example of the reactions is given in Table 1.

The results are of some interest in that they suggest a way of finding individual properties in human blood, namely, with the aid of immune sera against the blood of animals. As an analogy may be cited the demonstration of differences in sheep erythrocytes with immune sera for human A blood.[3] The reactions described, although of moderate intensity only, were obtained with immune sera produced at different times. Whether these observations may possibly lead to a method suitable for routine work is still under investigation.

* Reprinted from Proc Soc Exper Biol Med 43:223 (1940) with permission of The Society for Experimental Biology and Medicine, New York, NY.

[1] Landsteiner, K. and Wiener, A.S., J. Immunol., 1937, 33, 19.
[2] Wheeler, K. M. and Stuart, C. A., J. Immunol. 1939, 37, 169.
[3] Andersen, J., Z. f. Rassenphysiol., 1938, 10, 104.

TABLE 1

	Bloods (all group 0)									
	Type M				Type N			Type M, N		
	1	**2**	**3**	**4**	**5**	**6**	**7**	**8**	**9**	**10**
Absorbed immune serum	+	+	+	0	0	+	+	+	0	+

Technic: Immune serum for Rhesus blood diluted 1:10, absorbed with half volume of sediment of blood 4. One drop each of absorbed serum, cell-suspension (2%) and saline used. Readings after 2 hours at room temperature. Positive agglutination designed by + sign.

An Incomplete Antibody in Human Serum*

R. R. Race

From the Medical Research Council, Emergency Blood Transfusion Service

A study of the properties of mixtures of different types of human anti-*Rh* sera has led to the recognition of what appears to be an incomplete antibody. The research arose out of a suggestion by Prof. R. A. Fisher that this technique might throw some light on the problem of antibody absorption.

Human anti-Rh serum of the type called by Wiener "standard" agglutinates red cells of the gene Rh_1 and also those of Rh_2. "Anti-Rh_1" serum agglutinates the former cells but not the latter[1,2]. If, however—and this was the observation that started the present work—cells of the genotype Rh_2Rh_2 or Rh_2rh are added to a mixture of these two sera, the expected agglutination due to the standard anti-*Rh* serum does not occur. It was then found that the sera need not be mixed, for if the Rh_2 cells are suspended in anti-Rh_1 serum—which causes no agglutination—and after a few minutes are separated from the serum, washed and re-suspended in saline, then these treated cells can no longer be agglutinated by standard anti-*Rh* serum.

In January of this year Fisher drew up the following formulation of the relationships found in the Rhesus factor, designed to distinguish the three categories, antigens, genes or allelomorphs and antibodies for which provision must be made in a satisfactory notation.

The three forms of allelomorphic antigens are arbitrarily denoted by *C, c, D, d, E, e,* chosen to avoid confusion with any symbols so far used. The antibodies with which these react are denoted by corresponding Greek letters. These single letters refer to antigens and their corresponding antibodies only. Every gene of the system seems to be associated with a selection of three antigens from these three pairs. The system thus predicts an eighth allelomorph, Rh_z, which could not be recognized in a single individual, but could be identified in a favourable pedigree. It also suggests the possibility of two more antibodies not yet known reacting with *d* and *e* respectively.

* Reprinted from Nature 153:771 (1944) with permission of the publishers and the author.

Name of serum:	Anti-Rh_1	St	Anti-Rh Standard	Anti-Rh_2	Not yet found	
Antibody present:	Γ	γ	Δ	H	δ	η
Genes						
Rh_z CDE	[+]	[−]	[+]	[+]		
Rh_1 CDe	+	−	+	−		
Rh_y CdE	[+]	−	[−]	+		
Rh' Cde	+	−	−	−		
Rh_2 cDE	−	+	+	+		
Rh_0 cDe	−	+	+	−		
Rh'' cdE	−	+	−	+		
rh cde	−	+	−	−		

Those reactions not yet determined serologically are given in brackets.

	Rh_2 cells untreated				Rh_2 cells coated with anti-Rh_1 serum			
Serum dilutions	1/1	1/2	1/4	1/8	1/1	1/2	1/4	1/8
Anti-Rh_1 serum (Γ)	−	−	−	−	−	−	−	−
Standard anti-Rh serum (Δ)	+	+	+	+	−	−	−	−
St serum (γ)	+	+	+	+	+	+	+	+
Anti-Rh_2 serum (H)	+	+	+	+	+	+	+	+

Wiener[1] has supposed that the presence of the Rh_1 gene results in there being two "partial antigens" on the red cell (*C* and *D* of the table), and our recent work with *St* and other sera seems to make three parts necessary to the total antigen resulting from the Rh_2 gene, namely, *c*, *D* and *E*.

It is only one of these three antigens in the Rh_2 cells, called *D* in the table, which is being blocked by the anti-Rh_1 serum. *E* and *c* are left uncoated and ready for agglutination.

The coating of this same *D* antigen in Rh_1 cells can be demonstrated, but first it is necessary to remove the agglutinin (Γ) in the anti-Rh_1 serum for Rh_1 cells. This was done by absorption of the serum by $Rh'rh$ cells which remove the agglutinin but not the coating factor, since these cells contain *C* but not the coatable antigen *D*. With the resulting absorbed serum, cells of the genotype Rh_1Rh_1 can be coated without agglutination confusing the result. There is no blocking of the antigen *C* in Rh_1 cells.

Absorption with untreated Rh_2 cells diminishes the agglutinin titre of standard anti-Rh (Δ), anti-Rh_2 (H) and St (γ) sera. Absorption with coated Rh_2 cells diminishes the titre of anti-Rh_2 and St sera but not that of standard anti-Rh serum. Thus, absorption experiments confirm that in Rh_2 cells it is only the antigen *D* which is being blocked, *E* and *c* being left free.

The coating factor may be looked on as the standard anti-Rh serum antibody (Δ), which can combine with its appropriate antigen, but is defective in that it is not a suitable partner for the second stage of the antigen-antibody reaction which results in agglutination of the cells. It may be called an incomplete antibody (Δ'). Varying salt concentrations failed to produce agglutination of the coated cell suspensions, so did variations in the pH.

The incomplete standard anti-*Rh* antibody (Δ') has been found in good strength in four anti-*Rh₁* sera (from *Rh* negative mothers) and in a weak amount in our remaining anti-*Rh₁* serum (from an *Rh* negative mother). With the removal of the incomplete antibody, these five sera gained no fresh agglutinating range; they did not, for example, then behave as anti-*Rh'* sera. In other words, there is no complete standard anti-*Rh* serum antibody present which is being masked by the presence of the incomplete form of this antibody.

One standard anti-*Rh* serum in our collection contains the incomplete antibody (Δ') as well as the complete agglutinin (Δ). Titration results with this serum and *Rh₁* or *Rh₂* cells had previously given what was a puzzling and unique appearance—weak reactions, with intervening negatives, continuing up to a high dilution (1/1,000). Preliminary absorption with, say, *Rh₂* cells removes the incomplete antibody leaving the normal antibody, which now gives strong reactions up to the same titre with more of the same *Rh₂* cells. It seems as if the incomplete antibody wins the race for antigen.

Incomplete antibodies have been looked for but not found in three *St* sera, four anti-*Rh₂* sera, one standard anti-*Rh* serum, two sera from normal *Rh* negative donors, and eleven sera from normal *Rh* positive donors. The appropriate antigen *D* in all cells so far tried has been coatable; the cells were *Rh₁Rh₂*(1),*Rh₁Rh₁*(3),*Rh₁rh*(3),*Rh₂rh* or *Rh₂Rh₂*(6) and *Rh₀rh*(1). The incomplete antibody can be removed from serum by appropriate but not by inappropriate (for example, *rhrh*) cells, nor by saliva from an *Rh₁Rh₁* *A₁B* secretor. Heating to 56 °C. all the sera involved made no difference to the reactions.

I do not know of any similar phenomenon in haemagglutination or haemolysis. The inhibition by normal serum of the tissue haemolysis of red cells recently reported by Magraeth, Findlay and Martin[3] is evidently of a very different nature. The inhibitor described by these workers was not species specific, whereas the incomplete antibody now being described is specific down to one antigen.

In bacterial agglutination a more striking resemblance is found in the agglutinoid phenomenon studied by Shibley[4]. The most obvious differences are that agglutinoid was made by partial heat denaturation of the serum and showed itself only as a zone of inhibition followed in higher dilutions by normal agglutination; whereas in the anti-*Rh₁* sera, which had not been heated but stored at $-20°$C., all the standard anti-*Rh* antibody was in the incomplete form while all the anti-*Rh₁* antibody was in the complete form. The behaviour of anti-*Rh* sera, heated to 65–70 °C., is now being investigated.

Very recently a sixth anti-*Rh₁* serum has been found, locally. The incomplete antibody was present in good strength immediately after taking the blood.

REFERENCES

1. Wiener, *Proc. Soc. Exp. Biol. and Med.*, 54, 316 (1943).
2. Race, Taylor, Cappell and McFarlane, NATURE, 153, 52 (1944).
3. Magraeth, Findlay and Martin, NATURE, 151, 252 (1943).
4. Shibley, *J. Exp. Med.*, 50, 825 (1929).

Rh Gene Frequencies in Britain*

R. A. Fisher and R. R. Race

From the Department of Genetics, University of Cambridge
and The Medical Research Council, Emergency Blood
Transfusion Service

The genetics of the Rhesus factor have turned out to be so complex and our understanding of it has advanced so rapidly that it is difficult for many to arrive at a clear picture of the situation now substantially established. The notation has been frequently changed, and we feel that only a notation which designates unambiguously the antibodies, the genes or gene-complexes, and the antigens with which these antibodies react can avoid widespread confusion. In Table 1 we set out such a notation suggested by Fisher[1] which has been in use in this laboratory for about eighteen months. Six of the gene designations here adopted are due to Wiener[2], but for the antibodies his notation seems arbitrary. While Cappell's names[3] such as anti-C, anti-D, anti-E and anti-c are unambiguous, Wiener's do not seem satisfactory since, for example, the 85 per cent reacting serum is called anti-Rh_0, whereas besides Rh_0 it reacts with the genes Rh_1, Rh_2 and Rh_z. In the designations here used, on the contrary, Δ or anti-D indicates that the serum reacts with an elementary antigen D present equally in the gene complexes of Rh_0, Rh_1, Rh_2 and Rh_z, as shown in Table 1. (For the remainder of this communication the h will be omitted from Rh.)

The red blood cells of 927 Cambridge transfusion donors have been tested for agglutination with the four types of anti-Rh sera called Γ, Δ, H and γ in this notation. The sample was selected only in that the majority of the bloods were Group O or Group A. Tests on an unselected series of students not included in this total suggest that the distribution of the Rh groups is independent of the ABO groups.

This total of 927 does not include the first 154 persons to be tested with the four sera[4]. It is probable that the frequency of $R''r$ in this sample is by chance too high, for Stratton[5], examining a much larger sample with antisera capable of recognizing $R''r$, found only 41 out of 4,924.

* Reprinted from Nature 157:48 (1946) with permission of the publishers and the authors.

243

TABLE 1

English % positive	Anti-bodies	R_1 CDe	R_2 cDE	r cde	R_0 cDe	R″ cdE	R′ Cde	R_z CDE	(R_y) (CdE)
70	Γ	+	−	−	−	−	+	+	[+]
85	Δ	+	+	−	+	−		+	[−]
30	H	−	+	−	−	+	−	+	[+]
80	γ	−	+	+	+	+	−	−	[−]
65	δ	[−]	[−]	[+]	[−]	[+]	[+]	[−]	[+]
96	η	+	−	=	[+]	−	+	[−]	[−]

The following gene frequencies are an approximate maximum likelihood solution of the data above:

Γ Δ H γ	Total	Per cent	Most frequent genotype in group
− + + +	113	12.19	$R_2 r$
+ + + +	126	13.59	$R_1 R_2$
+ + − +	326	35.17	$R_1 r$
− − − +	137	14.78	rr
+ + − −	183	19.74	$R_1 R_1$
− − + +	12	1.29	R″r
− + − +	23	2.48	$R_0 r$
+ − − +	6	0.65	R′r
+ + + −	1	0.11	$R_1 R_z$
+ − + +	0		R′R″
+ − − −	0		R′R′
+ − + −	0		$(R_y) R'$

Although R_1, R_2, r, etc., are conveniently spoken of as genes, they probably each represent a short strip of chromosome involving three loci, there being two alleles at each locus, C-c, D-d, and E-e.

The interaction of the *Rh* genes and antibodies as they are now known are shown in the following table:

R_1	CDe	43.61 per cent
r	cde	37.90 ″
R_2	cDE	12.80 ″
R_0	cDe	3.05 ″
R″	cdE	1.70 ″
R′	Cde	0.81 ″
R_z	CDE	0.13 ″
(R_y)	CdE	probably no more than 0.005

Fisher's theory of three linked loci[1] was based on the reactions within the enclosure[4], particularly on the antithetical reactions of the 70 and 80 per cent sera. The reactions outside the enclosure were predicted by the theory; those in brackets are yet to be confirmed serologically. Mourant[6] has found η. The description of the serum[7] giving some of the reactions predicted[8] for δ now proves to have contained an error, and it is clear that the serum being described was an example of γ, and cannot now be identified as δ.

If the elementary antigens c, d and e are separable genetically, crossing-over between them will occur, though doubtless rarely. From this point of view it is to be noted that the three common heterozygotes,

R_1r	33 per cent
R_1R_2	11 $''$
R_2r	10 $''$

making together 54 per cent of the population of Britain, are all doubly heterozygous in the elementary antigens and would produce, by crossing-over, respectively,

$$R_0 \text{ and } R',$$
$$R_0 \text{ and } R_z,$$
$$R_0 \text{ and } R''.$$

It is tempting to think that these four rarer genes in the British population are maintained by such occasional cross-overs, especially since this view would explain the fact that R_0 is nearly as common as the rarer three put together and that R_y, the only remaining combination, could not be produced by cross-overs in these common genotypes, and is in fact known to be exceedingly rare, no certain case having been discovered.

Since the frequency ratio of R'' to R_2r, representing a cross-over between d and e, is considerably larger than the ratios of R' to R_1r (cross-over c/d) and of R_z to R_1R_2 (cross-over c/e), it may be inferred that the order within the chromosome is such that c lies between d and e, or possibly that c is a small inversion or deletion. Of the heterozygotes capable, on this view, of producing R_y, only the triple heterozygotes need be considered. Of these, R_1R'' has a frequency of nearly 1.5 per cent but could only produce R_y by a double cross-over; R_2R', with a frequency 0.21 per cent, would produce it by the cross-over c/e; and rR_z, with a frequency 0.1 per cent, by the cross-over c/d. If, then, the antigenic combination R_y is not exposed to especially severe counter-selection, we should expect it to be maintained by crossing-over in the two latter cases with a frequency which may be provisionally estimated at 48 per million.

Using this estimate, we may assess the chance of discovering this eighth missing allelomorph from the frequencies of the genotypes bearing it in combinations which can now, or will later, become recognizable. Thus $R'R''$, with a frequency of about 277 per million, is serologically indistinguishable from rR_y with a frequency of about 37. Only about 1 in 8 of this rare phenotype would then contain R_y. The genotype $R''R_z$, 44 per million, is indistinguishable from R_2R_y, 12 per million. This phenotype can now be distinguished by Mourant's serum as η-negative, but in the absence of δ is still confounded with R_2R_z, about 330 per million. Finally, $R'R_z$, 21 per million, is indistinguishable from R_1R_y, 42 per million. Both absolutely and relatively, this is the most likely group in which to detect R_y, but at present it is indistinguishable from the larger δ-negative group R_1R_z. These three groups must contain more than 90 per cent of the R_y genes, and their rarity, combined with the difficulty hitherto experienced in isolating them, fully explains the fact that R_y has not yet appeared in any unequivocal case.

REFERENCES

1. Race, NATURE, 153, 771 (1944).
2. Wiener, SCIENCE, 99, 532 (1944).
3. Cappell, GLASGOW MED. J., 125 (Nov. 1944).
4. Race, Taylor, Cappell and McFarlane, NATURE, 153, 52 (1944).
5. Stratton, ANN. EUGEN., in the press.
6. Mourant, NATURE, 155, 542 (1945).
7. Waller and Levine, SCIENCE, 100, 453 (1944).
8. Race, Cappell and McFarlane, NATURE, 155, 543 (1945).

Chi-Square Table

CRITICAL VALUES FOR THE CHI-SQUARE DISTRIBUTION

P

df	.99	.975	.95	.90	.75	.25	.10	.05	.025	.01	.001
1	—	0.001	0.004	0.016	0.102	1.323	2.706	3.841	5.024	6.635	10.827
2	0.020	0.051	0.103	0.211	0.575	2.773	4.605	5.991	7.378	9.210	13.815
3	0.115	0.216	0.352	0.584	1.213	4.108	6.251	7.815	9.348	11.345	16.268
4	0.297	0.484	0.711	1.064	1.923	5.385	7.779	9.488	11.143	13.277	18.465
5	0.554	0.831	1.145	1.610	2.675	6.626	9.236	11.071	12.833	15.086	20.517
6	0.872	1.237	1.635	2.204	3.455	7.841	10.645	12.592	14.449	16.812	22.457
7	1.239	1.690	2.167	2.833	4.255	9.037	12.017	14.067	16.013	18.475	24.322
8	1.646	2.180	2.733	3.490	5.071	10.219	13.362	15.507	17.535	20.090	26.125
9	2.088	2.700	3.325	4.168	5.899	11.389	14.684	16.919	19.023	21.666	27.877
10	2.558	3.247	3.940	4.865	6.737	12.549	15.987	18.307	20.483	23.209	29.588
11	3.053	3.816	4.575	5.578	7.584	13.701	17.275	19.675	21.920	24.725	31.264
12	3.571	4.404	5.226	6.304	8.438	14.845	18.549	21.026	23.337	26.217	32.909
13	4.107	5.009	5.892	7.042	9.299	15.984	19.812	22.362	24.736	27.688	34.528
14	4.660	5.629	6.571	7.790	10.165	17.117	21.064	23.685	26.119	29.141	36.123
15	5.229	6.262	7.261	8.547	11.037	18.245	22.307	24.996	27.488	30.578	37.697
16	5.812	6.908	7.962	9.312	11.912	19.369	23.542	26.296	28.845	32.000	39.252
17	6.408	7.564	8.672	10.085	12.792	20.489	24.769	27.587	30.191	33.409	40.790
18	7.015	8.231	9.390	10.865	13.675	21.605	25.989	28.869	31.526	34.805	42.312
19	7.633	8.907	10.117	11.651	14.562	22.718	27.204	30.144	32.852	36.191	43.820
20	8.260	9.591	10.851	12.443	15.452	23.828	28.412	31.410	34.170	37.566	45.315

INDEX